THE SEPARATING SICKNESS
Maʻi Hoʻokaʻawale

STIGMA

This book is about the stigma of leprosy in Hawaii and how sick Hawaiian people were treated. But today it might also be about the stigma of AIDS, or SARS or the Bird Flu. Anywhere. It is a book about fear. Fear of pandemic, and fear of sick people. Fear of the unknown. Same stigma, different diseases. Diseases with no quick cures or fixes. In the future, Public Health policy could very well be the same with other diseases as they were with leprosy in Hawaii. Mandatory isolation. This book is about fear and the disgrace, shame, and imprisonment of sick people, and what those sick people experienced. It is painful to read some of their descriptions. Let us hope that in the future, compassion, understanding and assistance to those affected by disease will prevail. Let us not lose our humanity in the face of fear.

Ted Gugelyk

Publishing History

First Edition, Social Science Research Institute
University of Hawaii, 1979

Second Edition, Maʻi Hoʻokaʻawale Foundation, 1985

Third Edition, The Separating Sickness Foundation
(Ma'i Ho'oka'awalei) 1996

Fourth Edition, 2005, Copyright by Ted Gugelyk, Milton Bloombaum and the
Separating Sickness Foundation, Published by Anoai Press.
Printed by Darnsutha Press, Bangkok, Thailand

ISBN: 0-9653971-0-6

Cover Design by John Shklov

Front Cover: Father Damien's grave at
                    St. Philomena Church, Kalaupapa

Back Cover: The Visitation room at Kalaupapa

Distributed by Ted Gugelyk
3349-Anoai Place
Honolulu, Hawaii 96822
USA
Contact by Email: kukui@lava.net

THE SEPARATING SICKNESS
Ma'i Ho'oka'awale

by

Ted Gugelyk and Milton Bloombaum

Excerpts from interviews with exiled leprosy patients at Kalaupapa Settlement, Molokai, Hawaii, as part of the Social Aspects of Leprosy Research Project, University of Hawaii—Milton Bloombaum, Principal Investigator; Ted M. Gugelyk, Co-Principal Investigator.

Published by the Separation Sickness Foundation

Dedicated to the Maʻi Hoʻokaʻawale Foundation and to leprosy patients and their families, in Hawaii and elsewhere; all those who were exiled because of society's reaction to the disease, but especially to the people of Kalaupapa.

ACKNOWLEDGMENTS

Funds to support the research from which these interview excerpts were drawn came from a grant under the Biomedical Sciences Research Program, awarded by the Office of Research Administration at the University of Hawaii, and from a grant from the Lani Booth bequest administered by the Department of Health, State of Hawaii.

Funds to facilitate publication were provided by the Maryknoll Fathers.

Special acknowledgments to the Kalaupapa Patients' Council and the patients of Kalaupapa, whose acceptance of the authors made the research and Maʻi Hoʻokaʻawale possible.

CONTENTS

Photographs follow page 90

v

PUBLISHER'S FOREWORD TO FIRST EDITION

When the manuscript for this volume was first submitted for publication by the Social Science Research Institute, the question of whether it represented social science "research" was raised. There were no surveys, no statistical analyses, and no control group comparisons. In short, none of the classic social science research methodologies were employed beyond that of the standard face-to-face interview.

However, the absence of such rigorous social science methods does not lessen the value of this work. Given the subject matter, the only appropriate methodology was that which was used: elicitation of social history from the only sources available, the residents of Kalaupapa.

The story presented in this volume is a moving one, containing deep insights into human feelings. There is much to be learned from these survivors of what is now seen as a bleak chapter in the social history of Hawaii, one which we hope will never be repeated.

The narratives of the residents of Kalaupapa can lead to better understanding of our fellow man for all of us, social scientist or not. If that is the goal of social science research, then this work is right on target.

D. M. Topping

PREFACE

This is a people's narrative--a biographical recollection, retrospective and contemplative, personal, painful, and at times angry--about what it means to be a leprosy patient in Hawaii in the early 1900s and today. But a people's history depends on the personal oral recollection of an experience. Accuracy is the extent of the genuineness of an experience. Here, documentation is individual perception, footnoted and punctuated by the accuracy of one fact--the experience of having been diagnosed and confined as one with the Ma'i Hookaawale--The Separating Sickness (Leprosy).

Perception of one's past influences perception of one's present and future. Since Kalaupapa people have not had an easy life ("we came up the hard way"), remembrances of difficulties endured makes them careful. Shy and weary of strangers, skeptical of administrative intents, policies and politicians, they wish one thing above all--a secure home at Kalaupapa. They also wish to be left alone--by photographers, tourists, and the other curious, including writers such as myself. "It's hell answering your questions. We try to duck people like you!"

Yet social scientists and journalists are a curious and perseverant breed. They always investigate the lives of minority groups, be they minorities like Blacks or Chicanos, or leprosy patients. I am interested in the latter. Leprosy patients voluntarily confined, and for the most part isolated, on a little peninsula on the island of Molokai, in Hawaii. The peninsula is called Kalawao, and their "hometown" is Kalaupapa. Leprosy patients have been sent to Kalaupapa for 103 years, from 1866 to 1969. They were sent there involuntarily--against their will--as a public health measure to combat the spread of the leprosy bacillus, and that is where Father Damien served the patients from 1873 to 1889 and brought worldwide attention to the little community. Involuntary confinement lasted in Hawaii until almost 1970, but similar confinement of leprosy patients occurred throughout the world. Before the innovation of sulfone drug therapy in the 1940s, millions of persons were confined or imprisoned. In

Hawaii, many thousands were affected. Kalaupapa is filled with the graves of those confined there in the past, and this book contains some of the stories of the 128 patients still remaining at Kalaupapa. Now they remain there by choice. They talk about their feelings and what it was like to be imprisoned at Kalaupapa. Why do they elect to remain in the community since they are now free to leave and reside elsewhere? Are they bitter about their lives, angry at society or the government about the treatment they have received historically and in the present? These are personal narratives, maybe oral histories, individual reflections on lives lived in confinement.

The Method of Research

Perhaps social scientists are reformers at heart. My reformist tendencies were established long before I developed an interest in sociology. Thus, I take comfort in Mark Twain's words, "always do good. It will surprise some and please others." I have tried to do good in these interviews. That is, present as accurately as possible the social effects of leprosy affliction--from the patient's point of view. The intent of this partial transcription of field notes, then, is to present subjectively, from the point of the patient, the internal personal meaning of having been involuntarily isolated at Kalaupapa, although legally they are now free to live elsewhere should they wish to. Thus, it is the patient's definition of the situation that is presented, but this definition is reformist-oriented, because the patients suggest improvements for the leprosy control program in Hawaii, and appear skeptical about the administration of their future. This study is not, then, an objective and empirically sophisticated policy analysis. It emphasizes the subjective. Although other methods of social science research stressing the more "scientific" approach will be used in later publications concerned with this study, including policy analysis, this portion of the work attempts to define reality by asking the person afflicted with leprosy, "What is it like, being a leprosy person?" I think that question is important, because perhaps, there is no final certainty in social science, no criteria for what is real, other than an individual actor's subjective meaning attributed to an experience. So, some human experiences with leprosy are documented here in the patients' own words and hopefully an interpretive understanding of the social aspects of leprosy affliction will be reached. In this work, I claim no interest in prediction, final truths, or experimental techniques. I do hope, however, that this accounting will be useful.

Background of the Study

My interest in Kalaupapa goes back to 1967. Part of my Master's work in Sociology at the University of Hawaii concerned itself with preliminary demographic research at the Kalaupapa leprosarium. Results of that research were published with Milton Bloombaum in the Journal of Health and Social Behavior in 1970. My current interest in Kalaupapa is part of the Social Aspects of Leprosy Research Project, also with Dr. Bloombaum (Principal Investigator). The project is a cross-cultural investigation of the phenomena of leprosy stigma in the State of Hawaii. Thus, early 1967 investigations were concerned with the transition of the Kalaupapa leprosarium from a community of patients involuntarily confined and isolated to a group voluntarily confined as "cured" patients. Conclusions were that reverse isolation was due to prolonged tenure in the institution, disfigurement, and stigma imputed by the patients to the general community.

Current research, the accounting of which is partially and briefly presented in this work, is more concerned with self-esteem and degree of depressive affect among the Kalaupapa patients. Thus, standardized social-psychological instruments have been administered to almost all of the patients in residence at Kalaupapa. In addition, in-depth interviews of patients have been conducted eliciting information about stigma perceived by patients, the understandings and attitudes towards their disease, and summarizing patient biographies and their lives in general. A small portion of those interviews (the subjective perception section) are presented in this volume. The Kalaupapa questionnaire contains over 110 separate items, and has taken over two years to administer to the residents of the community. Individual interviews have lasted as long as six hours. Most of the findings from Part I of our research are still in the process of being analyzed. In addition, Part II of our project is concerned with a cross-cultural State of Hawaii survey of attitudes towards leprosy and selected other diseases. This survey will provide us a basis for ascertaining the relationship between general community attitudes towards leprosy and those of the patients. The researchers assume one of the major problems in international leprosy treatment is the one of public awareness and acceptance of patients, before and after cure.

The Present Study: Entree into the community and building patient confidence

There is difficulty in doing social science research at Kalaupapa. Although leprosy stigma may be a major problem in treatment, locally and internationally, and public acceptance of leprosy patients may be limited in some places; similarly, patient acceptance of the curious researcher is also limited. The problem of entree into the community is a major one, as it is in all kinds of research concerned with minority groups. Of course, a few Kalaupapa residents are always eager to speak to newspaper reporters or researchers, however, the majority of Kalaupapa patients do not wish to be researched or considered as subjects. Indeed, many patients consider themselves to be subjected or disenfranchised, held in check historically and presently in a kind of quasicolonial status by the Hawaiian government. Thus, the political, ideological, and ethical concerns of the 128 Kalaupapa patients made it imperative that the social scientist be sensitive to the community needs as perceived by the patients. In addition, although research clearance to work at Kalaupapa was first obtained from the administrators of the community leprosarium (the Hawaii State Health Department), final approval rested with the patients themselves. Clearance had to be obtained from the elected representative body of Kalaupapa patients, the Kalaupapa Patients' Council.

The Kalaupapa Patients' Council reviewed the research, and finally participated in the formulation of the research questionnaire administered to community residents. This was only fair. The Health Department also had input into the research, as well as contributed some monies to the project

4

from the Lani Booth Estate. But the patients' input was special. Not only did they suggest research questions I would have never thought of, they also facilitated the inception and acceptance of the project within the community.

Thus, the research project was introduced and sanctioned at a community meeting with almost half of the residents in attendance. The Chairman of the council personally introduced me to each member of the community—the introductions and the first sixty interviews took about a year and a half. We did not rush our work within the settlement.

Patient cooperation with the research project also highlighted some other aspects of my work within the Kalaupapa community. That is, the moral and ethical dilemma I faced as one of the researchers. That is, to what extent does a researcher remain neutral, detached, and objective in the face of conflicting community needs and expectations? In some instances, perceived community interests were diametrically opposed to Hawaii State Health Department policy stances, and patients asked me the questions, "How will your research help us?" and, "Will your work be used against us?" In answer to the above, I say neutrality is not possible, although objectivity is. If detached neutrality is to mean overlooking community needs and perceived community concerns expressed by a majority; if neutrality is detachment in the name of a higher abstract principle of theoretical order, then such neutrality is exploitation. Kalaupapa people are not open to exploitation. Yet, objective fact finding is possible, if the researcher remains sensitive to various concerns which transcend immediate political expediency—be it the expediency of the policy makers or patients.

So, this research is not neutral, but it is objective, in that the tone of statements made by patients is typical of the Kalaupapa community. A kind of research bargain has been struck. Our final research results will be distributed to both patients and to the State Health Department. Hopefully, such information will be beneficial both to the patients and to the Department and will contribute to the enlightened administration of the leprosy treatment program in Hawaii.

As stated in one of our preliminary publications concerned with a health policy question our research has touched on (the closure of Hale Mohalu Hospital in Honolulu over the strong objections of almost 90 percent of the Kalaupapa patients), "when it comes to the consideration of the social as opposed to the medical and/or physical care aspects of patient life, there is no special reason to believe that any non-patient's views . . . deserve greater consideration than the views of the patients themselves." (The Star, Vol. 37, No. 5, May-June, 1978).

In this collection of retrospective personal narratives, then, various patient points of view are expressed. Together, they give us a feeling of what it is like to be a leprosy patient in the Hawaii of 1978.[1]

A Note about Leprosy--the Disease

Although leprosy has been recognized for over two thousand years, it was not found to be caused by a microorganism until 1873, by Dr. Gerhard Armauer Hansen. Leprosy, sometimes called "Hansen's Disease," is caused by Mycobacterium leprae, a member of the same family of organisms in which is found the cause of tuberculosis. It is a chronic communicable disease, thought to be transmitted directly from person to person, but only a small proportion of those exposed to an infectious case actually come down with the disease.

Leprosy is a disease of the peripheral nerves, but it also affects the skin and other tissues, especially the mucosa of the upper respiratory tract, the eyes, muscles, bones and testes. The two major forms of leprosy are called "lepromatous" (a progressive form in people with little resistance to it) and "Tuberculoid" (a self-limited form in those with more resistance). It is the Lepromatous form which causes skin lesions containing large numbers of bacteria, thus facilitating transmission of the disease to others. If left untreated, Lepromatous leprosy grows steadily worse, infecting internal

6

organs and the respiratory tract. Gross physical disfigurement also may occur in the advanced stages. The Tuberculoid form is more localized and benign, primarily affecting the skin and nerves. Here bacteria are sparse and present very little hazard in transmission. Usually spontaneous healing occurs in the tuberculoid form, but often with some permanent nerve damage. At Kalaupapa, older patients originally mandatorily confined with the tuberculoid form have attested to the spontaneous healing phenomenon. Because of this, some patients feel an error was made in the original diagnosis leading to confinement.

Among populations with some resistance to the disease developed through many generations of experience among Europeans and Asians, the tuberculoid form is more common. But among populations with little resistance, as among the Hawaiians of the 1800s, the more severe lepromatous form was usually contracted. It is estimated that ninety percent of the world's population has a natural immunity to the disease, and persons working with leprosy patients rarely contract the disease. But the disease does have a three to fifteen year incubation period before the first signs of it appear, and many afflicted patients claim no previous contact with known leprosy patients. It is thought that children are more susceptible to the disease than adults. Transmission often occurs within families, probably because in most societies children are most likely to be touched by relatives.

Since the 1940s, leprosy has been readily treated using drugs of the sulfone family. The disease can be "arrested" and patients rendered noncommunicable, therefore for those reasons isolation and confinement of persons with the illness is no longer necessary. Those who now remain in isolated places, like the patients at Kalaupapa, remain there by choice. But the seriousness of the disease and its effects are not past history. The World Health Organization estimates there are about fifteen million cases of leprosy worldwide, and less than twenty percent receive regular treatment.

Today, leprosy is found mainly in underdeveloped countries in Africa, Asia, Central and South America. In the United States, there are approximately three thousand known

7

cases, primarily in Texas, Louisiana, Florida, California and Hawaii. In the United States approximately 350 persons are treated at the U.S. Public Health Service Leprosarium at Carville, Louisiana. Carville is the only continental U.S. institution devoted exclusively to the treatment and research of leprosy. It was there that sulfone drugs were successfully introduced in 1941. In Hawaii, there are approximately 440 registered patients receiving treatment. Of these, about 128 of them are older patients at Kalaupapa, institutionalized before 1969, when the decision was made to do away with long confinement of treated lepromatous cases. The other 310 are tuberculoid patients, or new lepromatous ones, treated on an outpatient basis or in community hospitals. There are approximately thirty new cases of leprosy diagnosed in Hawaii each year, over 90 percent of whom are immigrants from Asia, Southeast Asia, and Pacific. The number of new cases found among Hawaii-born people is approaching zero.

Kalaupapa—The Community[2]

The residents remaining at Kalaupapa are vestiges of an international public health policy which physically and socially isolated people thought to be carrying the disease of leprosy (sometimes called Hansen's Disease--after Dr. G. Armauer Hansen, a Norwegian who discovered and isolated the mycobacterium leprae in 1873). Although Kalaupapa was established in Hawaii in 1866, other total institutions or leprosariums like Kalaupapa were established throughout the world. Compulsory segregation legislation was passed in Norway in 1885; in New South Wales in 1890; in Cape Colony, South Africa in 1892; in Japan in 1900; in Ceylon in 1901; and in Canada in 1906. In addition, two of the most famous leprosy colonies are Culion, in the Philippines, established in1901; and Carville, established by the United States Public Health Service in Louisiana in 1894. Kalaupapa, then, may have been a kind of international public health model for the isolation and containment of the disease, and for those who carried it.

For thousands of years, however, victims of leprosy have been treated differently than those suffering from other

8

diseases. Historically and traditionally, isolation of leprosy persons was the norm. Some societies even killed leprosy victims, but most cast them off to some isolated mountain or island. Before the innovation of sulfone drug therapy in the 1940s, public health practices for dealing with the disease were not too different than those of centuries past. But in the 1800s the means for dealing with the disease became more formal. In Hawaii, and elsewhere, laws were established legally enforcing isolation of leprosy victims. "Laws touched upon marriage and divorce, estate and income taxation, claims against estates, absentee ballotting, employment rights and State pensions of patients, fishing rights in waters off Kalawao, separation of infants from mothers, penalty for concealing persons with leprosy, rights and duties of kokuas (helpers), the oath of loyalty, the practice of medicine, the sentence of convicts . . . clearly, the legal, social and medical history of leprosy in Hawaii is an integral part of the historical fabric of the Islands."[3]

There is evidence early Hawaiians feared the Board of Health and mandatory isolation at Kalaupapa more than the actual affects of the disease of leprosy. Often, friends and family readily hid infected persons within households, rather than surrender them to a life of banishment at Kalaupapa. Yet, between the sixteenth and seventeenth centuries, a period of European exploration and colonization, Western governments were faced with the biomedical uncertainties of the etiology and epidemiology of a disease primarily endemic to non-Western people. Leprosy was envisioned as a foreign "non-white" disease--as strange and exotic as the newly contacted cultures. The early establishment of colonies like Kalaupapa may reflect an early social conception of the illness that is uniquely Western, and with instrumental functions as a defensive response. Governments feared a pandemic spread of leprosy throughout western territories and possessions. So, many "total institutions" like Kalaupapa were established.

Western attitudes toward the disease were affected by the biomedical uncertainties of its origin, spread, and cure. Perhaps leprosy was considered a disease of inferior people, and therefore associated with low standards of living. In

9

addition, biblical references to leprosy helped create a public conception of it with uncleanliness and defilement. This taint of uncleanliness and "moral impurity" gave a stigma to those unfortunates afflicted with leprosy and to the colonies to which they were sent.

There is evidence of cross-cultural differences regarding the degree of stigma associated with the disease. It was observed that "native Hawaiians possessed an absolute fearlessness and absence of any disgust for the disease in its worst form."[4] Thus, the Hawaiian people feared the compulsory banishment and rough treatment by European and Hawaiian public health agents more than the disease itself. In fact, there was a high rate of intermarriage between the Hawaiians and the Chinese, who had given them the "Mai Pake" or the Chinese sickness. Also, "in countries where leprosy is highly endemic, stigma is not necessarily pronounced, whereas among Western nations where the prevalence of leprosy is low and historically debatable, a presumption of extreme stigma has emerged."[5]

The establishment of early Western attitudes, such as hopelessness of cure and revulsion to the disease, was reinforced by Christian missionaries such as the martyr, Father Damien, who worked for sixteen years among leprosy patients and died of leprosy at Kalaupapa in 1889. Believing that leprosy was incurable, Western clinical medicine abandoned leprosy patients and left them to the grace and mercy of dedicated Christian fieldworkers. Acting in the "extraordinary service" of Christ, Western missionaries began a worldwide service to leprosy colonies in 1874. To this day, working with Leprosy Patients is a field still dominated by Christian (church) agencies.

Leprosy was thought to be a "totally maximal illness," thus the negative social and emotional responses to the disease. Dr. Olaf Skinsnes' (1964) hypothetical disease model expressing the ultimate in physical disablement and social revulsion might apply to leprosy. Thus, a totally maximal illness would: (1) be externally manifest; (2) be progressively crippling and deforming; (3) be non-fatal and chronic, running an unusually long course; (4) have an insidious onset; (5) have a fairly high endemicity, but not be epidemic; (6) be associated with low standards of living; (7) appear to be incurable, and (8) have a long incubation period" (Gussow and Tracy, 1970).

After 1946, the innovation of prophylactic treatment by drugs of the sulfone family, along with Penicillin and Mycin, made leprosy cease to resemble a maximal illness. The psychological effects of the disease could be arrested. Similarly, physical deformity resulting from the disease could in some cases be corrected by plastic surgery. However, although the Mycobacterium leprae could be controlled physiologically, the negative social-psychological concept of the disease may not lend itself to rapid abatement. In time, the Hawaiians, too, grew to fear the disease. According to the World Health Organization, perhaps no other disease causes such a reaction in the community and so much distress and unhappiness to patients and their families. This anxiety may follow leprosy patients and relatives throughout their lives and cast a shadow over their families and professional and social activities. Fortunately, the situation is gradually changing. Nevertheless, prejudice still persists to a degree that is not found with any other disease." [6]

It has been over thirty years since the introduction of sulfone therapy, but there has been a continuous resident population at Kalaupapa and other communities like it; but there has been a dramatic shift in the character of confinement. Prior to 1946, virtually all residents of the Molokai colony were legally quarantined as bacteriologically active patients. In 1866 there were 141 involuntarily confined residents; in the 1890s about 700; and in the early 1900s over 1,000. By 1966, twenty years after therapeutic relief became available, the community had 162 patients. However, out of this number only thirty-one were classified as active. In December 1968, the population consisted of 141 individuals of which 20 were active. In February 1975, there were 149 residents of which a similarly small percentage were active. By August 1978, there were 128 patients voluntarily in residence at Kalaupapa.

Therefore, a significant number of "cured" patients elected to remain in the total institutional setting, for most it had become a community, and most of all, it had become a home. Even when they were eligible to return to the general community; they voluntarily confined and isolated themselves from the society to which they might have returned. Today, their median age is close to sixty, having resided half a lifetime or more in confinement, and most are partly deformed and scarred. There are also lesser numbers of Chinese, Japanese, Filipino, Samoan, and other ancestries residing in the settlement. There has evolved a type of reverse isolation among the patients, reinforcing a culture different from mainstream Hawaii.

Most of the residents at Kalaupapa are Hawaiian or part-Hawaiian (almost 60 percent). Yet within the State of Hawaii they make up less than 20 percent of the total population and may be considered a displaced minority within their homeland. As with the American Indian, Kalaupapa may represent a type of reservation, a special place for maintaining alienation from the larger culture of Hawaii. The Hawaiian reservation of Kalaupapa, the maintenance of alienation and a different culture, are forms of a socially-sanctioned protection of identity and beliefs which serve not only to protect from the stigma, shame and discreditability of association with the "outside" world (which leprosy patients attest to suffer in association with outside people), but more importantly the maintenance of alienation and a different culture may represent the preservation of a "last Hawaiian place." The culture of differentness may be like the culture of originality which existed before the coming of the Western discoverer, the trader, missionary, administrator, and the coming of the "Mai Pake" itself. Although Mai Pake took away something precious from them as did the trader and missionary, unlike the latter, Mai Pake may have also given something back. And that is a final home, a place of belonging, to the community or extended family (ohana) and the land (the aina). That is very important to Kalaupapa people today. That is why they wish to remain at Kalaupapa (in the face of a rapidly diminishing population) and at their old treatment facility in Honolulu, Hale Mohalu (closed down in 1978 by the Hawaiian State Health Department). They are familiar places, home, a place earned after a lifetime of banishment and ostracism.

Perhaps Hawaii's leprosy victims symbolize leprosy victims throughout the world, and their reflections about society's treatment of them may be a valuable footnote to the history of the disease. State law mandates Kalaupapa people may remain in the community as long as they wish. Ninety-five percent of the residents wish to remain there for the rest of their lives, but they are the last of their kind. Sulfones made that possible. There will be no future generations. There have been no new admissions to the settlement since 1969.

In this book, the patients speak of their lives, their pasts, and their hopes for the future, at Kalaupapa. It is precious land, the Kalaupapa land. Although the people at Kalaupapa will be allowed to remain, the community has become smaller each year and use of the peninsula remains unsettled. There are possibilities of a national park there, or maybe a State of Hawaii or County of Maui Park (in consort with the current residents). There is also talk--most unpopular among Kalaupapa residents--about resort development. However, one resident missionary has hopes for a Pacific research and treatment center there in keeping with the community's history and record of dignity, in the face of human suffering.

The newly-established fifteen member Kalaupapa National Historical Park Advisory Commission has been mandated by federal law to examine the possibility of turning Kalaupapa into a national historical park. The alternatives and future use of the land are yet to be decided. In the midst of the studies, alternatives, debates, and uncertainties, here, then, are some of the life stories from the few people remaining at Kalaupapa.

Ted Gugelyk

NOTES

1. The interviews were conducted individually between May 1977 and March 1978. They are, then, transcriptions of my field notes, edited for style and standard English usage. Nevertheless the final interview statements have been read back twice to each patient to confirm the accuracy of experience and intended tone of the narrative.

2. Portions of this section were first presented in a paper entitled "The Social Aspects of Leprosy: A Working Paper," by M. Bloombaum and T. Gugelyk, presented to the session of Medical Sociology, annual meeting of the Pacific Sociological Association, Sacramento, California, April 1977.

3. Thomas Hitch, <u>A New Look at Leprosy in Hawaii</u>, Health and Community Services Council of Hawaii, 1969.

4. Z. Gussow and G. S. Tracy, "Stigma and the Leprosy Phenomenon: The Social History of a Disease in the Nineteenth and Twentieth Centuries," <u>Bulletin of the History of Medicine</u>, 44 (September-October), pp. 425-499.

5. <u>Ibid.</u>

6. World Health Organization, WHO Expert Committee on Leprosy, <u>Fourth Report</u>, WHO, Technical Report Series, No. 459, Geneva, 1969.

INTRODUCTION

The patients of Kalaupapa live in a setting perhaps best designated as "total institution," e.g., a place of physical and social isolation. The by now well-known institutional processes leading to self-mortification, institutional identity, and (in part) situationally determined perceptions of other patients, staff, state administration, and outside members of the general community have been operative over a very long period of time. We are attempting to record the lifelong social experiences in relation to leprosy of each patient. Indepth focused interviews individually conducted by Mr. Gugelyk, co-Principal Investigator for this project, have taken from one to six hours. In the larger project we are interviewing leprosy patients in settings other than the Kalaupapa settlement, as well as leprosy workers and a sizable probability sample of the general population living in the state of Hawaii. We hope ultimately to be able to view the experiences and attitudes of patients in the light of both their perceptions of attitudes towards diseases among members of the general community, and the objectively measured general community attitudes towards diseases. Our project is difficult, time consuming, and expensive. We have taken measures in the midst of expressed difference of opinion and political controversy between Kalaupapa residents and health administrators in Hawaii's Department of Health to maintain our objectivity, to retain the good will and cooperation of both patients and health administrators, and above all to direct our research activities in such a way as to preserve the main purposes and anticipated long-range benefits of this research. Various circumstances have forced delays and we are as much as a year behind our original time schedule; anyone who is familiar with the vicissitudes of ongoing social research in the field will not find this unusual.

When we arrived at Kalaupapa in order to present our request for cooperation and approval from the patients' council (after having negotiated approval and cooperation from the Health Department) for this research project, we were met with a question put to us that we had not anticipated. Certainly we were prepared to answer any and all questions regarding the scope and purposes of our project, and we were prepared to alter certain aspects on the basis of the reactions of the patients' council. But we were not prepared for the first serious question to come up, viz., "Are you going to spend the night?"! This was not only the first question but the first clue to uncovering events which had meaning for the patients. As it happened, we had planned to stay overnight at the settlement because we thought that we needed the time in order to get a feel for the place and to talk informally to several patients and staff. Had we not (fortuitously) so planned, I fear that our acceptance by the patients' council and ultimately by the entire patient population would have been more difficult than it was, or at any rate would have taken longer. The sad fact of the matter is that historically there have been those among the health administrators responsible for the leprosy program, and the welfare of the patients who themselves would avoid any sort of personal contact with the patients, in some cases even after the introduction of effective procedures to arrest the progress of the disease and to render it noncommunicable among those so treated. Of course there also were those among the administrators who sought contact with the patients and valued them as human beings. Presumably the larger general community of our state harbors some whose behavior is governed by fear and ignorance, as well as some whose behavior is more rational. Do the leprosy patients at Kalaupapa have a right to expect that the staff that administers their program and serves them will be favorably disposed when it comes to personal contact? That is a question that our research project is not likely to answer; however it is because of the project that we can bring such a question to light, and to suggest that the general community be prepared to deal with it.

The patients have a stake in this research project; as I see it the main issue is not different from that faced by any of us in the course of our lives. When the time comes to die, what is it that we can leave that will turn out to have been a contribution to the lives of others? The leprosy patients at Kalaupapa can leave something which is to them, and to them alone, unique; they can leave for others the records of how society banished them, of how they were treated while in a

16

state of social isolation, of their reactions throughout, and, particularly, during the period subsequent to the introduction of effective treatment. It is a record of the human experiences of a very special population--a population who because of their disease and because of the public reaction to their disease have lived lives that the rest of us haven't. What we learn from this record of human experience will at its best serve to enrich our own lives and those of the generations succeeding us. We will learn to be exceptionally sensitive to the idea of social banishment; we will learn, above all, that human dignity is worth preserving.

Of course, the patients want more than to have their records preserved. They want to be assured and reassured frequently that Kalaupapa will be theirs as long as they want it. They want to be involved in deciding what is to be done with the peninsula after they are all gone. When their numbers drop to 100, 50, 30, even 10 they will want continued assurance that their living arrangements will continue to be meaningful in human terms. Right now they want Hale Mohalu at Pearl City returned to them as a place for treatment, visits, and in some cases residence on the island of Oahu.* They want to be a force in their own lives, and to move consciously away from the essentially paternalistic treatment of which they have been the recipients since 1866. There undoubtedly are other things that they want. Will they get everything they want? Should they get everything they

---

*On January 26, 1978, the Hawaii State Department of Health officially closed the Hale Mohalu facility at Pearl City, on the island of Oahu, and transferred the few resident patients to a newly designated for leprosy treatment section at Leahi Hospital behind the slopes of Diamond Head some 15 miles from the Pearl City site. Many patients resident at Kalaupapa, on the island of Molokai, protested the move and have been in continuous occupation of the Pearl City facility. It is important for the reader to be aware of this struggle between the leprosy patients and the State in order to understand some of the references appearing in certain interview excerpts.

want? If they get everything they want does this not mean that any institutionalized population (such as retardeds, mental patients, prisoners, or the blind) will by precedent have a claim on everything they want? What it boils down to is whether this particular group of leprosy patients, having experienced at the hands of society physical and social banishment, the loss of family and friends thus entailed, and all the other consequences, both good and bad, of their having been diagnosed as afflicted with leprosy, are now felt by the members of the general community to be so deserving as to constitute a case for "affirmative action." Our research project is not likely to be able to answer these questions in the scientific manner expected by us and of us. However, we can and by virtue of our project, do bring such questions into the public arena for general consideration. We do provide data on the lives of patients heretofore unavailable, and data on the attitudes of general community members formerly only imputed to them by others. All this is not here provided in this short book--it awaits the completion of the project and publication of the monograph which will constitute the main report.

We have been interviewing at Kalaupapa for many months now and as of the end of 1978 have completed ninety interviews with patients. Many of the statements were made by patients in response to open-ended questions such as:

"Are you bitter?"
"How did people treat you on the outside?"
"Where do you want to spend the rest of your life?"
"Where have your worst experiences been?
"Do you think people on the outside are prejudiced against you?"
"What is the worst thing about being a leprosy patient?"
"What is the best thing about being a leprosy patient?"
"Do you want to continue receiving treatment at Hale Mohalu or Leahi" Why?"
"Why do some people avoid getting treatment for leprosy?"
"How does the Department of Health administer Kalaupapa and Hale Mohalu?"
"Does your family visit you here? How often?"
"Do your children visit you? How often?"

"Do you want your family notified when you die?", etc. Since all of the interviews have not yet been done, and the overall analysis of data awaits completion of the remaining interviews, as well as the other parts of the project, we are not yet in a position as researchers to write the final report. Still, some of the answers to questions such as those listed above have been so very rich in their human content, we have decided to provide a limited number of excerpts from a selected set of completed interviews. We feel it may be important to do this at this point in time (that is, before the project is completed in its entirety) because events in relation to leprosy treatment, mainstreaming philosophy, and emerging consciousness on the part of the general community of how to deal with special populations are moving so rapidly.

A few comments of a methodological sort seem in order. First, a caveat as to the interpretation of the material presented here. It should be obvious to the reader that these excerpts cannot, from a scientific point of view, be treated as the sum total of patient experiences at the Kalaupapa settlement. Neither do they provide a sound basis for generalizing to the responses of all patients. It is clear from the excerpts presented that a wide range of diversity exists; the diversity, in fact, is considerably wider than can be here shown from the selected interviews. Yet, there is strong stuff here; the reader will be educated as to the feelings, perceptions, and attitudes of some patients, and will be able to form a concept regarding a type of life outside the ordinary experiences of persons living in conventional settings.

The interviews were done on an appointment basis, one or two, or perhaps three interviews in a day; the task is very demanding. It was possible for the interviewer to spend usually one day each week at Kalaupapa. This means that the method of this phase of our research most probably should not be characterized as participant observation, which some social scientists would regard as desirable for these circumstances. We felt that if the interviewer became a part of the everyday life at Kalaupapa, he would come to be perceived as belonging more to one segment of the community than to another, and that this would work so as to take away from the willingness of some to respond openly and honestly. An anthropologist who goes into a small community for ethnographic purposes typically will remain in the community on a continuous basis, select a limited number of key informants (perhaps five or six), and check his interpretations of informants' statements by observing behavior directly. Since we are more concerned with the past experiences of the patients, and with the current interpretations of the patients, things that are not necessarily visible in the overt behavior exhibited by patients, we feel that interviewing on a nonparticipant basis is the desirable method. Of course, some direct observation of patient behavior by both of us at Kalaupapa and elsewhere was done and constitutes in part the fund of general knowledge we have gained about leprosy-related phenomena.

There are twenty-five interview excerpts in this book, some only a paragraph long and some going on for several pages. The first, entitled "Am I Bitter?" illustrates a more or less typical attitude common to many patients. Getting leprosy is just bad luck, no one is to blame, and one ought to be thankful for what one has. The excerpt shows acceptance of, perhaps resignation to life's situations. The second excerpt entitled "Self Respect: Dignity and Pride" points up the problems of secondary diseases and side-effects connected with the use of effective medication. The meaning of self-respect for this patient inheres in taking pains to be clean for his medical examination. Since he was blind he was not in a position to know whether he had gravy stains on his shirt and was therefore additionally dependent upon other patients. Here is personal courage and dignity in the face of adversity. The third, entitled "My Family: They Hookai (reject) Me," describes the circumstances associated with this patient's diagnosis and removal. Her expressed feelings of having been rejected serve to suggest why many patients are reluctant to leave what they experience as the relative safety of Kalaupapa in order to return to live in the general community. Number four is called "Leave Your Bones at Kalaupapa," and after providing a description of this patient's experiences in connection with diagnosis and removal shows the difficult time she had in accepting her mother's rejection and her children's refusal to respect her wishes in regard to the use of the word leprosy. But accept she did and her sense of self is connected with her own determination of where she will die. The next, "Why Did It Happen to Us Hawaiians?", serves to call attention to the fact that Hawaiians show a higher rate of contracting the disease than do other ethnic categories in Hawaii. The notion that leprosy may run in families comes through here, as does the fact that many nonafflicted who are in long-term, close contact with those who are do not themselves contract the disease. This patient reacts against institutional life; he resents that decisions for his own life are made by others and without reasonable explanation. He feels that his medicine is worse than his disease. This patient, whose life has been a marvel of independence, twelve times delivered his own children! He continues to struggle with the question of why it happened to the Hawaiians.

The sixth, seventh, and eighth excerpts, The Sterilization Program I, II, III, call attention to the fact that children are thought to be more susceptible to the disease than adults; the newborn were quickly removed from Kalaupapa. The sterilization program was instituted presumably to reduce the number of children born to leprosy patients. The voluntariness of the program seems to have been compromised by making submission a condition for getting approval for visits to Honolulu. There is mention of anger. In the second of these excerpts the patient views the sterilization as castration. The third patient relates that an alternative line of visit to Honolulu was for special eye treatment.

Interview nine has the surprising title "I Love the Word Leprosy." The informed reader knows that there continues to be controversy over the use of the term leprosy. But not in the mind of this patient who views the community at Kalaupapa as having given her life its fundamental meaning. She blames a kahuna for her disease and states that she contracted it while at Kalaupapa and was thankful she could stay. To her, the word leprosy sounds sweet! She is unhappy only that Kalaupapa has not been maintained as it was. "I Was a Guinea Pig," excerpt ten, relates the embittered story of a patient diagnosed at the age of ten. He expresses deep resentment over being used in medical experiments, and

21

regards new patients as lucky since effective treatment is available to them.

In "The Time Capsule," a patient relates that the worst thing for her was not bringing up her own children. Her deep spirituality provided comfort, but she wonders why patients always have an uphill struggle in getting a measure of human respect. She is fearful that Kalaupapa will be taken away; she views the staff as noncaring. There is resentment against what appear to her as the arbitrary decisions and actions of the authorities. In "Kalaupapa: My Home Town" the patient explicitly reveals that Kalaupapa is the basis for his sense of identity; Kalaupapa is paradise. He shows significant resistance to the idea that patients can be reincorporated into the general community. His own attempt in that direction failed for reasons he attributes to the old Board of Health. "From Dust to Dust" reveals general bitterness and anger towards the Health Department. He is not too happy about being asked to answer such personal questions as we have put to him. He relates that he was done out of a job for which he was trained. He wants the rights of leprosy patients to be recognized; he perceives a great deal of stigma in the outside community against leprosy. "I Became One of Them" details in encapsulated form the range of experiences and feelings of a patient who is frankly suspicious of the Department of Health. She questions why permits are necessary for family visits at Kalaupapa, given that Kalaupapa patients are themselves free to leave the settlement. She doesn't understand why her grandchildren cannot visit, and why those who are permitted to visit are limited to fourteen days. Yet in spite of her critical attitude, her overall perspective on life is quite positive; she remains close to her family and children. This patient brings up the point that prescribed medication is to some extent, in fact, controlled by patients rather than doctors; an arena for self-determination is thereby created and a considerable measure of responsibility is taken by some patients for their own bodily welfare. In "My Big Kalaupapa Family," a patient describes how important the settlement has been to him from the age of five. A period of unhappiness characterized his life when he was moved back to the general community, but he regained his happiness once more upon his return to Kalaupapa; his closest friends have been dying off and social

22

relationships are not now what they used to be. Without bitterness he notes that buildings, grounds, and programs have deteriorated from what they once were.

In "No More Family Ties," a blind patient points out that his blindness in his case was not due to leprosy. He perceives his life as having been unfortunate; he does not fix blame in any particular place. His tale reminds us that Orientals with leprosy suffer perhaps as much from the shame of the affliction as from the disease itself. Excerpt seventeen, entitled "This Place is Heaven," reemphasizes the point about shame. He regards having contracted the disease as putting his parents in a tough spot; his spirituality seems to help him maintain his positive perspective. Kalaupapa is "heaven" for him.

In "Akerameru," a patient goes a little more deeply into the difficulties of the social unacceptability of leprosy among Orientals. Leprosy spoils your ancestry. This patient feels both shame and bitterness, but is explicit in accepting her fate. For the remainder of her life she does not want to be mingled with nonafflicted people--she clearly prefers remaining at Kalaupapa. "That Wild Germ, Bucking Like a Wild Horse" emphasizes feelings about physiologically experiencing the disease, as well as the difficulties associated with separation from family. Here is a patient who feels good about not having been rejected by his family and lucky to be able to see his children, grandchildren, and great-grandchildren. Hale Mohalu for him has been important as a place where his family could visit with him. In the excerpt entitled "Love Could Not Overcome Fear," a patient who could have returned from Hale Mohalu to the general community describes the conditions under which she chose to reside at Kalaupapa. Her experiences with prejudice coming from her first husband and his family seem so vivid as to negate the ordinary meaning of our question about prejudice on the outside.

An unusually articulate patient undertakes to describe the differences between treatment available at the U.S. Public Health Service Hospital in Louisiana and treatment for

Kalaupapa patients in "I Paid My Own Way to Carville." He is very concerned about foot problems. He was a volunteer for horse toxin treatments which worsened his condition, although he has now overcome that. His independent analysis of his situation leading to his insistence on receiving treatment at Carville and even paying his own way pioneered the now available procedures for other patients in order to receive advanced treatment. This patient uses the modern term Hansen's Disease, a term strongly preferred by patients at Carville.

"The State Has Provided; I Am Grateful to Our Benefactors" presents a very positive view of the role of the Health Department. A detailed description of the circumstances surrounding detection of the disease and a period at the old Kalihi receiving station is followed by an account of this patient's attempt to make a place for himself at Kalaupapa. He views having been sent there initially as a punishment; his deep attachment to his religion helps him to make peace with his circumstances.

Not every source has to be an interview situation; here in the twenty-third segment we exhibit a letter translated by Ruby Johnson, Associate Professor of Hawaiian at the University of Hawaii. The story is told by a woman who went to Kalaupapa in order to be at the deathbed of her son, and to remove his cremated remains. Her granddaughter felt sufficiently moved to retain the account for the family genealogy.

"The Long Road" is a compelling account by a patient of his life since diagnosis. Against incredible odds he completed a university degree in 1978, and has high hopes for the future. He describes how the disease progressed in his case, and details the problems associated with being blind. His is a story of strength, will and independence.

The final interview excerpt entitled "Leadership" details some of the early life experiences of the Chairman of the Kalaupapa Patients' Council, as well as this patient's views on what it is like to stand up and fight for patient rights. Interestingly, his removal to Kalaupapa (and that of all the children at the receiving station) took place under the unusual circumstance of the Japanese bombing of Pearl Harbor in 1941; a quick decision was taken at least in part for the presumed benefit of the afflicted children who thereby would be protected from bombing and gunfire. Growing up in Kalaupapa for this patient was painful due largely to the disease itself, and when effective treatment became available for him in 1948, his life took a turn for the better. His early years led to a later level of maturity (personal, social, and political) that finds him taking major responsibility for the welfare of all the patients; he does this even though it would be personally better for him to be in Carville in order to receive special treatments. He is a remarkable man, unafraid to contend with power; he counts as his friends and supporters many legislators and others in high places. Here is a clear example of how a leprosy patient participates in the main stream of social/political life in the general community which is Hawaii.

This then is the range of human material here provided from our interview materials to date. Following are the selected accounts in the patients' own words, edited for clarification, the final version in each case having been read back to the patient and approved as to wording, sentiment, and tone.

M. Bloombaum

AM I BITTER?

Am I bitter that I contacted leprosy? No, I'm not bitter. I hold no grudges. It just happened. Just bad luck. We had no choice coming here, you know. They took us away to Kalaupapa fast. I was only seven, and I did not know what was happening. They came to get me at school. I think the teacher reported me to the Board of Health. They used to get ten dollars for each leprosy person they reported. First I went to Kalihi, then they sent me here. Oh, I missed my mommy. She came a few times to see me, but then pau, no more. She had other kids. I think they kind of forgot about me, but I got used to it. My parents <u>make</u> now, they are dead. I don't know where my brothers and sisters are. It all happened a long time ago. That's how it is. Who can you blame? You just thank God for what you have.

Male, Part-Hawaiian
Blind, Disabled
Age: 59
47 years at Kalaupapa

SELF- RESPECT: DIGNITY AND PRIDE

No, I'm not bitter about this disease. I have been here at Kalaupapa since I was twelve. Maybe I'm lucky. I never think about it too much. I get three square meals a day here. I get care from the nuns and the nurses. I have my talking books and I listen to my big band music. I still listen to my Glenn Miller and Artie Shaw records. I like that kind of music. You know, since they sent me to this place I have never stepped outside Kalaupapa except to go to the hospital in Honolulu--to Hale Mohalu.

Like the other patients, they caught me at school. It was on the Big Island. I was twelve then. I cried like the dickens for my mother and for my family. But the Board of Health didn't waste no time in those days. They sent me to Honolulu, to Kalihi Receiving Station, real fast. Then they sent me to Kalaupapa. That's where they sent most of us. Most came to die. So, I stay here. But one thing about this sickness, you get other problems because of it. It seems we all have to suffer, all through our lives--one problem after the other. Me, I've got the heart problem and stomach ulcers. I'm blind and I can't walk. Then I get side effects from the sulfone drug medicine. Still, maybe I'm lucky. In Kalaupapa, we are all in the same boat; we help one another. We are one family, all the same, with love in our heart ... with aloha for each other. Oh, we fight between ourselves, like in any family, but we are all in it together here. There is no where else for us to go.

You know, my worst experience was when I was already inside Kalaupapa. It was bad for me, especially because I knew my family suffered. After they caught me, they didn't stop with me. No. They nosed around my family. The Board of Health in those days was not confidential. The social worker was always looking for others in my family with the mai Pake. She used to go to people's homes and try and catch them by surprise. She came in an official marked car, driven by a chauffeur, dressed in a white gown. Terrible! She used to upset everyone, because the neighbors would know. The family felt shame. After her visits she used to gossip about my family saying things like, "they pilau (dirty)." The family—they wanted to forget me, and I don't blame them. My sister came here to see me, maybe twenty years ago. We lost touch with one another.

I don't know if people are prejudiced against me. I keep to myself here, and I try to keep my self-respect. When the doctor comes for the medical clinics, I try to make sure that I am clean before I see him. I know that is something the doctor appreciates. I want to please him. So, I take a shower or bath and try and make myself presentable. But sometimes, later, I learn that I had a spot of coffee on my shirt, or maybe some gravy. But I don't know that unless somebody tells me. They should tell me those things. Is that what you call self-respect?

(Two months after this interview, the patient died at Kalaupapa. He was buried by his fellow patients on the 4th of July.)

Female, Hawaiian
Partly Disabled
Age: 69
51 Years at Kalaupapa

MY FAMILY: THEY HOOKAI ME

They caught me when I was eighteen or nineteen. The Board of Health gave the neighbors ten dollars for reporting me. That was the policy in those days. One evening the Health Department inspector came to our house to examine me and pick me up. He said I had to go with him to Honolulu. If I said no, he would put me in handcuffs and drag me off. They threatened us that way. But I did not want to go, because I had this little boy who was my hanai boy. I loved him so much. But they said I would give him the sickness—mai Pake to the little boy—so for his own good, I went. They took me from _____ to Mahu-Kona, then to Kalihi Hospital in Honolulu. I was put on the ship Kaala. The same ship that later sank on the reef off Kalaupapa.

At Kalihi they kept us separated. Boys on one side, girls on the other. The next morning, I had my physical examination. I went into a room where six doctors waited. I was naked except for one white sheet they wrapped around me. Those doctors examined me, looked at the spots on my body. They talked among themselves for a few minutes, then they said I should return to the girls' ward. In a few days I received a large envelope with a letter in it. The letter had my name on it, and it said, "You have been declared a leper." So I was sent to Kalaupapa. I wish I still had that letter. I would show it to you, but it was lost in the tidal wave that hit Kalaupapa in 1946.

After that, I hate to tell you this, my family hookai (rejected) me. All of my relatives hookai me. They were sad and disappointed in me for getting this sickness, and after I got it they did not want me anymore. That's what the mai Pake sickness does. It hookai you from your loved ones. The name of leprosy is a fearful thing, they fear this disease. That's why they hookai me (separated me).

You know, when I was a little girl in _____, I saw this one sick man who lived like a dog. He lived in a shack. It looked like a dog house. At that time I didn't know it, but he was a man with leprosy. He lived in a lean-to, a little dirty place with a roof made of old boards. There were three sides to his shack, with one part open to the wind and rain. It was tacked on to the side of his family's house. His family lived in the big house and he lived in the dirty shack. He always stayed in that little place. He would hardly ever come out. He would just stay in there dirty and huddled up. When he wanted to eat, they would make him feed himself. He had to cook his own food. He had his own dish and fork. He could only eat after others finished eating. They did not let him touch anything of theirs. Sometimes they would allow him to use the kitchen stove to cook his food. But his family did not take care of him, and I used to watch him when I was a little girl. He was hookai too, just like I am now. Yes, I remember that poor man sleeping outside, all disfigured and twisted. I was just a little girl, and I did not know he had the leprosy sickness and that later I would get the same thing. I can say today, and I am ashamed to say it; but my family was no better than his.

After I was discharged, paroled or declared negative, I could have returned home. But my family asked me not to return home. They said not to come around. Do not try and live with the family. You know, when we die, our families will come to Kalaupapa and ask to see our graves. They also want to see our wills, but they will be surprised. I have no money.

Today, living on the outside, it's not so bad. But because of what happened to me with my family and friends, I don't feel comfortable outside. I have my own home here. This is where I will stay. Some of our people still have problems outside Kalaupapa. That's why they come back to Kalaupapa, even though they could live on the outside.

Female, Hawaiian
Married
Age: 70
46 years at Kalaupapa

LEAVE YOUR BONES AT KALAUPAPA

I was born on Maui, in the little community of Hana. I was twenty-seven when my mother noticed red spots on my body. I was married; I had two children. My family sent me to the doctor in Wailuku to look at the spots. Right away he knew. He said, if you go to Kalihi Hospital in Honolulu, they will cure you in three months. He promised me a cure for this disease. But my mother knew of this illness, and after the doctor examined me, she looked at me with sad eyes. She said, you have the ma'i hookaawale (the separating sickness). I think she knew I had the sickness before I went to see the doctor.

My mother did not want me to go to Kalihi Hospital. She knew more about the sickness than I did. Maybe she knew I would not be cured. So, she suggested I not show myself to anybody. She said, "Go hide. Hide inside the house. When someone comes to the house, run out the back door into the bushes on the mountain side." And I did that for three months. I went into hiding and the Health Department inspector did not find me. But, I had a husband and two children. There was so much crying over me, and I began to tire of the hiding life. I thought, I will try the cure. Maybe in three months I will get well. After all, the doctor promised. So, I left for Honolulu. My family told our neighbors I was going to visit relatives.

When I arrived at Kalihi Hospital, right away they put me into isolation on the women's side of the place. The next day they gave me a physical examination. My body was covered with red lesions--round rings with lumpy spots in the center, bumpy little spots. The doctors gathered around me while I stood there naked in the white tile room. I was cold, and I only had a sheet around me. The doctors said they

31

would give me the treatment. In those days, the only treatment was chaulmoogra oil. After three months, the chaulmoogra oil helped me. The red spots went down, but I never went home again. Even though the spots went down, they would not release me. Since they would not let me out of Kalihi, and because they were so strict there, I volunteered to go to Kalaupapa where there was more freedom. I found a new life at Kalaupapa, and my old life broke apart.

I remained in Kalaupapa for thirty years. I was finally paroled in 1966. My mother was still alive, so I wrote to her and told her I was finally cured. I could come home. After a long while, her letter came. She said, "Don't come home. You stay at Kalaupapa." I wrote her back and said I wanted to just visit, to see the place where I was born. Again, she wrote back. This time she said, "No, you stay there." You see, my mother had many friends and I think she felt shame before them. I was disfigured, even though I was cured. So, she told me, her daughter, "Don't come home." She said, "You stay right where you are. Stay there, and leave your bones at Kalaupapa." I don't blame her. I am more happy at Kalaupapa. This place is finally my real home. They take good care of me here.

I don't feel bad. I love this place now. These are my people. We are all together and we feel pity and love for one another. We try to help one another. I won't leave this place, because now I know people are still scared of this disease. As long as you are a leper, that's all, they still fear you. Chinese are most scared of this sickness, but Hawaiians are scared too.

The worst thing about having this sickness is having it. There is nothing good about it. I am no match for those outside people anymore. I am embarrassed by my scars. I am not fit to live with others. If they try to force us to leave Kalaupapa, I will commit suicide.

I hate the name leprosy. I like the name Hansen's Disease better. In the beginning, years ago, my children would write to me. On the envelope addressed to me, they would write Kalaupapa Leprosy Settlement. I did not like

32

that. I wrote to them and said, "Don't put that name leprosy on the envelope. Just put Kalaupapa." But when they wrote to me again, they put Kalaupapa Leprosy Settlement. So I stopped writing them, because they did not listen to me. We pulled away from one another because I don't want them to write to me with that name on the envelope. Even though I am here, they should have listened to me. I was still their mother. So, I will stay here. Like my mother said, I will leave my bones at Kalaupapa.

Male, Hawaiian
Widowed
Age: 81
67 years at Kalaupapa

WHY DID IT HAPPEN TO US HAWAIIANS?

My wife passed away at Kalaupapa. We celebrated our fiftieth wedding anniversary right here. She was a patient too. Like many of our people, we married one another inside Kalaupapa. Me, I am eighty-one now. Old man, eh? I have been confined since I was twelve. That is when they first diagnosed the sickness in me. I have been in hospitals for sixty-nine years--two years at Kalihi and sixty-seven years at Kalaupapa.

Things are not too bad with me. I am disabled, but it could be worse. I have no feeling in my hands and feet. My eyes are not too good either. Also, I have kidney trouble. But for my age, I'm OK.

They sent me to this place when I was fourteen years old. Like the other patients, they caught me in school. The teacher knew that I was what you call 'a contact.' You see, my ohana had leprosy through my father. My father died from this sickness at the old Kakaako Hospital in Honolulu. My brother died from this sickness here at Kalaupapa. So they all figured I was 'a contact.' I think they first found the sickness when they gave me the vaccinations in school. The teacher told the doctor that my father had the mai Pake, so I think she turned me in. People were so scared of this sickness. But I was lucky. Even though we had the disease in our ohana, my family never rejected me. Many people lost their families after they were sent here. That was real isolation then.

I think Chinese people were most scared of this disease, but the Japanese and Hawaiians were too. Today, maybe people are not so scared, but I know people still look at my hands when I go outside. I think people still fear us,

34

especially the older ones. But some folks look at my crab hands and think I had an accident. Plenty of us say that. What are you going to say to one stranger? I am a leper? The ones who recognize the signs of this sickness, those people shy away.

I don't believe you catch this disease from contact with leprosy people. Plenty people lived together in the ohana where one had it, and the rest never caught it. For instance, I know about one case that happened right here in Kalaupapa, and there were plenty like this one. There was one wife who loved her husband so very much. He caught the leprosy sickness. She knew they would send him away to Kalaupapa, so she wanted to catch it too. She loved him so much that she used to rub herself with the pus from her husband's leprosy sores. But she never caught it, no matter how hard she tried. Finally they caught him and broke them apart. They sent him to Kalaupapa. Later, the wife could not stand being apart from her husband, so she volunteered to come to Kalaupapa as a kokua (helper). That way, she stayed here with her husband until he died. There were so many cases like that, so I don't believe you catch the sickness from contact. That wife, she never caught it. Plenty other kokuas never caught it either. But the teacher turned me in. She thought I was a contact, and the law said contacts must be turned in and examined.

The worst thing about being a leprosy patient is that they shove you around like cattle. They take you here to die, and still they push you around--like this problem at Hale Mohalu. First they sent us to Kakaako, then to Kalihi, then to Kalaupapa, and now up to Leahi. Of course, we do get good things too. The government takes good care of me. I get my medical attention, my housing, food, like that. Sometimes, though, I think I may leave this place now that I am old. I think about my children and grandchildren, moopunas, you know? But maybe my family might be hurt if I get too close to them. Maybe people will talk. Maybe patients should live here with their own kind and not shame their families. But I wish the Health Department would let us be. We have been sent away enough. They move us from one place to another, against our wishes.

I think Hale Mohalu is a good place for us. It's easy for family to visit us there. We have privacy and plenty of space. It is like our home away from home in Honolulu. So close to shopping, friends, and I think we get good care there too. The people in Pearl City are used to us. The shopkeepers, they open their doors for us. In the beginning, they were frightened of us, just like other people. Maybe Leahi people will fear us, then we have to go through the same thing all over again. We are too old for that. No, I don't like Leahi. We have been shoved around all these years. Maybe, this is one more time of being shoved around. Always the same thing for us.

About my medicine--I never take it any more. Some other patients feel the same way. The medicine for this illness is no good for our kidneys. Me, I got well by myself. I think most people at Kalaupapa die from taking the treatment. They don't die from leprosy, but from the treatment! First, they gave us chaulmoogra oil. That killed people. Maybe with these other drugs the same thing happened. I think it's better not to take medicine. I don't take anything, except some Vitamin C. This sulfone treatment gives people kidney trouble, and they all die from that.

The worst thing about being in here is missing my children. I have twelve children and they were all born inside. Nine of my children lived. I delivered all of my own babies. They were all born inside Kalaupapa. Twelve children I delivered. The first few times, the midwife showed me how to do it. With the other nine, I delivered them myself.

You know, the babies that were born inside here were not allowed to stay with their parents. After the babies were born, the law said they had to be taken away to the baby nursery in Kalaupapa. They were afraid of the contact-- afraid the babies would catch the disease from their parents. But some of my children, I will tell you this, some of them I kept longer. Most times, the babies were born in the night. We kept everyone quiet so the administrators and nurses would not hear the baby being born. All my babies were born in my own home, right here. After I delivered the babies, we were so happy. I called the young girl patients and they would come running in the night to look at the newborn one. Everyone was so happy to see baby children. And us, we were so proud of our new babies, we had so much love. My babies stayed with me that way, longer than the law said they could. But my children never caught the sickness. We would try to keep the babies as long as we could, but most times, we kept them only until morning. Then we would carry them to the nursery. I didn't want any trouble with the administrators, or with the Board of Health. So we gave them up. That was the law. They allowed the children to live one year inside Kalaupapa nursery. There we could see them only through thick glass, but no can touch! Then after one year, they were removed. They were either hanai by family members, or "issued" out for adoption by the Board of Health.

It was so hard to give up your children like that, especially to the Board of Health. Seven boys and five girls we had. But three boys died in the nursery. They never took good care of them, yet they would not let us care for our own children, even when we knew they were sick. It was hard. You love them, and then they are taken away, just like we were taken away. But the children would never know us as parents. Well, I try to make the best I can of this disease. I have to like this disease. I have to make the best of it.

Tell me, why were there so many of us Hawaiians in here? Why did so many Hawaiians die in here? Why did it have to be that way, with us Hawaiians? Maybe when we were kids in school, maybe they gave us the wrong medicine, the wrong vaccinations? They caught me at vaccination time, like the others. Sometimes I think maybe they wanted to get rid of the Hawaiians. The plantations wanted our land, so they tried to get rid of us. I don't know. Our family had land on Maui in Hana, and the plantation there tried to take away our land. Who do I blame for this disease? I don't know. But why us Hawaiians?

Male, Portuguese
Widowed, Partly Disabled
Age: 73
57 years at Kalaupapa

THE STERILIZATION PROGRAM--I

About children, they didn't want us to have any. I don't have children, yet others inside here had plenty. They had a sterilization program inside Kalaupapa. Some patients will tell you it was a law. But there was no law, as far as I can remember, and I remember good about those things. There was a voluntary sterilization program. It was up to the patients if they were fixed. Some men say they were castrated, but I don't believe it. Ask them to show you to prove it. I think they get some things mixed up with age. But one thing for certain. They had a sterilization program. But they would ask us if we wanted to be sterilized. The doctor asked me back in 1941; he asked me if I wanted that operation. I said, "Doctor, if you want me to be sterilized, it's all right with me. It's up to you doctor." So he did. I think today you call it vasectomy? I don't know what they did with the women, but they did something. My wife, she never had nothing done to her. Sometimes the newcomers, the ones who only have been here twenty or twenty-five years, they may talk to you but they get their facts mixed up. They did not force us to get fixed up. We had a choice. But you know, we all remember that they tried to make a law that would force all leprosy persons at Kalaupapa to be sterilized. That upset and worried most everyone--every patient in here was upset. The sterilization program began around 1938, and I know they were still doing it up to 1942 or 1943. But there was one Territorial Senator, he introduced a bill into the Territorial Legislature asking for forced sterilization at Kalaupapa, for all patients over seventeen. Well, I think his Bill went into the wastebasket. So as far as I know, there were no forced sterilization. But we know that some people were thinking about making that kind of law.

38

Some of the other patients remember differently. For instance Mr. _____, who died here in the 1960s. He was an oldtimer too, and he had a college education. He was bitter. I remember he telling me, that they have taken everything out of us. They took us away from our families, they sent us here against our will, and even that wasn't enough. He told me not long before he died (we got together and talked story about the old times) that in 1938 they tried to promote that sterilization policy on us. Any patient who wanted to go to Honolulu for a visit, had to submit. Now you know, we missed Honolulu very much. Especially those patients who had children and family there. Those patients who were negative, were given a condition for permission to visit Honolulu. The Board of Health didn't want patients to have children. They felt children would get leprosy. So to prevent leprosy spreading from parents to children, they wanted us to submit to being made sterile, and also the men. Now Mr. _____, he was my friend; also said men were castrated. But I don't think he was actually castrated. But he said look, they took everything from us. What more do they want? They even wanted to take away your manhood and womanhood. Well, some men submitted. That's how desperate they were to get back to Honolulu and visit their family. But _____, he was one of the patients who fought that policy, and I think it was finally dropped around 1943, maybe after the Legislative bill was put in the wastebasket. But not before some patients submitted to the operation. But like I said, I think he was wrong. There was no official Board of Health policy about sterilization. They just tried to encourage us to get the operation done, but it was up to us. No one forced me to get it, but I did finally submit. I had that operation done right here inside Kalaupapa. Plenty patients though, went to Kalihi receiving station to get that operation done. But voluntarily, I think. Me--after I had that operation, I could go to Honolulu without too much trouble, since I was negative. But I don't think it was because of my operation. I think they get their facts mixed up, those others. Maybe they are just angry at their condition. Most of the women in here, they have been sterilized too. Plenty of them. Most of them.

Male, Portuguese
Age: 63

THE STERILIZATION PROGRAM II--
I SUBMITTED, AND I SAW MY ONLY SON

I wanted to go to Honolulu to visit my son. I could go on only one condition, to be made sterile. My son was only two and one-half years old. I had never seen him from the day he was born at Kalaupapa. They took him straight out. I wanted to see him because I loved him and I missed him. You want to see your child, especially your son. He was hanai, raised by family, and I got word he was sick. So I asked the administrators if I could go out and visit him. They said you can see him, but only if you are made sterile. They cut off my balls. You had no choice. That's the only way you could go, so I submitted and I went; I saw my only son.

No one can help. That's the only way you could go to Honolulu. As far as I can remember, that policy was in effect from 1938 to 1942. But I don't know when or how they stopped that policy. I think other patients just refused to submit to that operation after a while. But plenty others did submit. That's how desperate they were to get out of here.

Male, Japanese
Single
Age: 50
37 years at Kalaupapa

THE STERILIZATION PROGRAM III--
IT HAPPENED OFF THE RECORD

In the 1930s and early 1940s the only way you could get to Honolulu was either for eye problems to see one specialist, or medical problems, or to go to the sterilization operation at Kalihi receiving station. But it was voluntary, as far as I can remember. But that was the only way we could get out of here and visit Honolulu. Any other way to get there, I don't know. I don't speak to others about this too much. I used to see Kalaupapa people come to Kalihi--the majority for eye operations. But for sterilization, too. That's all I know; anything else about that I don't know; I can remember, quite a few of the women were sterilized there too.

These things have happened before--remember those two poor Black girls in Alabama? They were sterilized through the doctor's own decision--just about three years ago. Maybe those things still go on at Waimano Home, maybe at Kaneohe; I'm pretty sure those things happen, but how much, nobody knows. But here at Kalaupapa, this is a small place, you can't keep things like that secret. But these things happened a long time ago. I'm sure you won't find those things in the official record.

Female, Part-Hawaiian
Partly Disabled
Age: 44
33 years at Kalaupapa

"I LOVE THE WORD LEPROSY"

Who do I blame for my disease? I blame a kahuna. I
was cursed when I was ten years old. You see, my mother
was sent away to Kalaupapa. She had the sickness. My
father was left alone with me. Then he remarried. I did not
get along with my stepmother, so one kahuna wanted to hanai
(adopt) me. He asked my father if he could have me, but my
father said no. One day the kahuna came to our house and did
some kind of ceremony. The house was closed up; and the
parlor was made dark. And that kahuna man cut off a piece
of my hair and threw it into a pot of boiling water. I will
never forget it. A head rose out of the pot. I think from that
day on, they put a kapu on me. Nobody was to have me, not
my father nor the kahuna. After that, I started to have many
problems. From that day on a black curse stayed with me
until I came to Kalaupapa. In fact, it came to Kalaupapa
with me. They actually put one black cloth around my neck
and told me never to take it off. I wore it on the boat to
Kalaupapa. It stayed with me until the kahuna man died.

How was it that I was sent here? Like I tell you, my
mother had leprosy and she was sent to Kalaupapa when I was
still a baby. The doctor suspected I had leprosy when he
found a little red spot on my toe. Well, they immediately
thought I had the disease. So they didn't waste any time.
Since my mother had it, they told my father and stepmother I
would be sent off to Molokai. Actually we were very happy.
I was happy. I was looking forward to seeing my mother. I
also had one auntie at Kalaupapa, and one other relative too.
I was not happy with my stepmother, so I was looking forward
to being with my real mother.

After I arrived at Kalaupapa, oh, what a shock! I asked
for my mother, and the patients said, "Didn't you know?"

42

"What?" I asked. "She died," they said! What a shock! I cried and cried. She had died three years before I arrived and the Health Department did not inform my father. I wrote to my father to tell him the news. My mother was dead. She had not been here to meet me the way we hoped she would. My father became so angry at the Board of Health and the government, but it was no use. She was dead.

But I stayed at Kalaupapa. My foot healed up. They found out later that it was not leprosy I had after all. It was just a red spot on my toe. They took snips of that spot, did a biopsy of my toe, and still they found no leprosy. It all turned out negative. So they had sent me here for nothing. Since my mother had it, they thought I must have it for sure. That's how it was then. They sent you away real fast. Well, after that, the Board of Health wanted to send me back home to my father. But you know what, I did not want to go back home. I began to like Kalaupapa. So, my story starts.

Even though I was negative I wanted to stay at Kalaupapa. I did not want to go home. Two or three months at Kalaupapa was enough to show me that life was better for me inside than out. At home, we were poor. My stepmother did not treat me well. At Kalaupapa they treated me nicely. The nuns took care of me and the older patients showed me love. It was like I had one big family inside here. I was everyone's child. And there was so much food. For once in my life I could eat all I wanted. And there was dancing and singing in the old Hawaiian way. It was one big ohana. I grew to love Kalaupapa, and I still love it, even though it is different now that we are getting old. I had never been so happy.

So I wanted to stay, and I told the Board of Health I did not want to leave. The Board of Health said if I wanted to stay I had to face a board of five doctors. I had to sign five papers saying I wanted to stay at my own risk. They wrote to my father, and he had to sign papers saying he approved of my staying and that he understood the risk I was taking. I signed the papers also, even though I was just a child. My father approved, and that is how I got to stay at Kalaupapa. I loved the people at Kalaupapa, and I still do.

So you see, I caught the mai Pake after I came inside Kalaupapa. I don't blame the Board of Health for anything that happened. It turned out for the better. I took my own risk, and it was worth the risk I took. Two years later, when I started to show the real signs of leprosy, I knew I finally had it. I was so happy because I knew they could not send me out. Kalaupapa became my real home and I felt safe. I was so happy to get this leprosy sickness.

So, Kalaupapa gave me life! It was a good life, a real Hawaiian place. Nice Hawaiian music, dancing, and food. I had rather catch the sickness than go home to face my stepmother and our poverty. But then, when the disease took hold for real, I began to get sick a lot. I developed bad reactions, and I began to suffer for real, like the other patients. Yet, I still thanked God I got the disease. I didn't care how much I suffered, because I finally had a home.

Today, I am not sorry for anything that happened. I am happy to stay inside this place until I die. Outside I think there is still some prejudice and fear of this disease, especially here on Molokai--topside. Up there they all stare at us because of the way we look. We can tell by the way people look at us, how they feel about us. But I don't care. This is home. Let them continue to call us lepers or leprosy patients. I don't care for the other word, Hansen's Disease. I love the word leprosy! It sounds so sweet to me. It was in the Bible, and God healed the lepers, so why should we change the word? So you see, I am still happy. Nothing will make me move from Kalaupapa. No, money will never buy me out of the settlement, even though the Board of Health may offer to buy us out. I will stay here until I die, and I will be satisfied. The only thing wrong is that this place is getting run down.

Male, Part-Hawaiian
Partly Disabled
37 years at Kalaupapa

I WAS A GUINEA PIG

My uncle turned me in. He was so afraid of this sickness. Actually his own wife had it--my auntie. It was she who took care of me when I was a little boy. When she showed the signs of the sickness, they took me away from her. When my uncle saw I had the same signs, well, he turned me in. Can you imagine that? My father had much hate for my uncle after that. My father had been treating me with Hawaiian medicine at home. He took me to medical <u>kahunas</u> for help. I was ten years old. I had red spots on my face and some numbness in my fingers.

Even with the sulfone drugs, this illness gets worse. It knocks me down more. The new medicine doesn't help make your feeling come back in your nerves. It doesn't help your crab-twisted hands; and my club feet and legs still have no feeling. As I grow older, it grabs hold of me that much more.

One of the worst things about this illness is what was done to me as a young boy. First, I was sent away from my family. That was hard. I was so sad to go to Kalaupapa. They told me right out that I would die here; that I would never see my family again. I heard them say this phrase, something I will never forget. They said, "This is your last place. This is where you are going to stay, and die." That's what they told me. I was a thirteen-year-old kid.

The worst thing about being a leprosy person is that it deprived me of my happiness. I am not happy if I am one leper. I cannot live like other people live. I cannot do what other people do. I cannot get a good job. I can't have a good married life. I cannot have children. And when I go outside, even some old friends, how strange they look at me. Old friends show no pity. They only show a kind of scary feeling of me. So I don't want to go outside because of my

45

appearance. I know, when I touch something on the outside, sometimes others will not touch it. They shy away. That is why we stay among our own people, our own kind, and try and enjoy the life we have left. Here, among our people, we understand one another.

Truly, the worst thing about this whole program is how they used us children for guinea pigs. They used to experiment on us, against our will. They injected us with different kinds of medicine. They also used to "nose trip" us. We could not refuse. They said we were minors. If we did not cooperate, they would punish us kids. No can resist that "nose trip." They would stick one applicator stick up each nostril. That way they would force open the nose, since the nose was blocked up with mucus. They put opium on the stick to soften up the tissue, and shove the stick all the way up our nose. Then, they would take some metal instrument and pull out the applicator stick from deep inside the nose passage. With the stick would come the stuck mucus, tissue, and plenty of blood. Boy, that used to hurt. Every day they did that to me for two years. I could not resist. Every day I would bleed. That's why my nose is like it is, broken down and flat. For two years they slowly broke away the bridge of my nose. Because of that experiment I had almost constant bleeding for two years. That experiment did more harm than good. Look at me today--I'm the loser. I can't face other people. Other new patients are lucky, because later the new drugs came. They didn't have to go through what we did.

I only leave Kalaupapa about once a year. I like to meet friends. But I don't go to their homes. We meet in public places. I think people are afraid to let you into their homes.

Am I bitter that I contracted leprosy? Yes, I am very bitter. I think, why me? Why did I have to suffer? But I can't blame anyone for this illness. It just happened. But I do blame the doctors who used me as a guinea pig.

When I die, I don't want my family notified. I am alive now. Why don't they come to see me when I am alive. When I die, what's the use? It's too late. Now is the time to show care.

Female, Part-Hawaiian
Partly Disabled
55 Years of Age
42 years at Kalaupapa

THE TIME CAPSULE

The best thing about this disease is that it gave me my own home inside Kalaupapa. The worst thing is that I was not able to care for and bring up my children. That is my biggest regret. I could not be their mother. My children were born inside, but we hanai them. My mother raised my children. I see them once or twice a year. But they are grown now.

One thing about Kalaupapa. We help one another. To help others is so important. A lot of our people are self-taught. They learn something, then pass it on to others. Since we help one another, it makes us more aware about the importance of giving.

I am not bitter about my life or about this disease, because I believe in God. I have faith. What will be will be. What it was with me, it was. I am seeking a spiritual religion, something personal. All of us, we are all God's children. My husband and I, our faith in God is strong; God is in our home. We do not practice religion as a habit, without meaning--we love God in our own way. We believe God is everywhere. You can pray anywhere, even in the closet, and God will listen to you. What is important is to reach out to others less fortunate than we. You know, I think we live in one time capsule. I mean, our struggle today, the struggle of leprosy patients, is no different than the struggle of Father Damien. He had to struggle, and we have to struggle. But since the sulfone drugs, our struggles have been made easier.

But that is it, one time capsule. The same problem, over and over again. Why can't people understand our suffering? Look at me. No fingers, no feeling in my hands; I have a kidney problem, my eyesight is going, everything is going, yet they don't understand what we have gone through.

47

Since we were young children we have suffered. Yet, the authorities say we have too much! We struggle just like during the time of Father Damien. Maybe there is no change in people's attitudes or feelings towards us. How can they be so insensitive to our feelings and needs? Always it is the same ... first they moved us to Kalihi Receiving Station, then to Hale Mohalu, then to Kalaupapa, and now to Leahi. Where else do they want to place us? Forty-two years ago we were young, but now that we are growing older, more deformed and crippled, we can't take any more changes. No more moving from one place to another. Finally, the Governor of Hawaii said he would let us stay and they passed a law for us to stay. But I know, little by little, they are trying to get us out of Kalaupapa. Look at the run-down condition of the buildings. The time will come when they will try to get us out of here. They want the land. Even though they promised we can stay until the last one of us die, we know as our numbers decrease, they will make us move again. The day is coming!! Every few years they disturb us patients There is an apprehension among our people especially the older folks who have been here most of their lives.

They tell us Leahi is better for us. The move is for our own welfare. But the best medicine would be for them to leave us alone. We don't need that kind of help. They should try to heal the person. If the patient is not happy, if he is depressed, forced to make new adjustments again and again, he will not be a well person. That way, he may get sicker. They tell us Leahi is a better facility. Better buildings, facilities, service, like that. But if the patient is unhappy in being moved, over and over again, all the medication given to him will not help. If he is unhappy, he will not stay well. What is important for us patients is privacy and security. Peace of mind.

So I say, the authorities should try to do more to make the patients happy. They should do less to make us unhappy. Bring happiness, not sadness to our people. We need a caring staff. People with heart who can see the needs of our people. Not everything involves money. Simply caring, listening, and feeling wanted and respected as a human being, is important. It's just not good being shunted around because we have leprosy. We are grateful for what we have, but don't take what little we have away.

Male, Portuguese
No Visible Disfigurement
Age: 49
34 years at Kalaupapa

KALAUPAPA: MY HOME TOWN

When they sent me to Kalaupapa, it's not like I was one stranger coming to some strange place. No, not then and not now. When I was fifteen they sent me here, but I already had six family members inside Kalaupapa. The sickness is in our family. Besides me, there was my younger brother, my sister, two uncles, and my father. My father died inside this place. You might say, Kalaupapa is my home town.

It's strange that you should interview me today. This is my anniversary. Today, June 8, makes thirty-four years I have been inside this place. As far as I am concerned, I want to be buried inside Kalaupapa. No, I won't leave. I don't want to trade paradise for hell. At one time, it was hell inside. Now the hell is outside Kalaupapa.

We have all had hard times, both inside this place and outside. Me, I have felt prejudice against me. In the hospitals, by the hospital staff and by other patients, and outside from the general public. The Health Department, they always tell us, why don't you go out? You are still young, they say, go out and try to make a living outside. They seem to think it's better for us outside, but I don't think the public is ready to accept us. They try and put pressure on some of us younger ones to go outside. They want us to leave Kalaupapa and get a job. But let me tell you, I tried that, and I tell you, no more!

Me, I was a welder. I have a welding diploma from the old Honolulu Technical School, and I did have one job outside. I tried to make it outside. But you know what happened. I never got a fair shake! I never had a chance to make it outside. I didn't defeat myself, the old Board of Health

49

defeated me. That not only happened to me, it's not only me I am talking about, but other guys also.

Back in the 1950s I was declared negative and paroled. I found me a job and I was paying my own way in Honolulu. I left Kalaupapa and I wanted to make a go of it, like other people, on the outside. But something unbelievable happened. The social worker from the Board of Health came to my work place to check up on me, like I was one criminal. She told my boss, she said, "Did you know he is one leprosy patient from Kalaupapa?" I never told my boss. I was negative. I didn't have to tell nobody where I was from. I wanted to be independent, and I didn't want to scare nobody. But she came around, and she scared the boss and the other guys I was working with. They fired me. How come? I was negative. But because I was from Kalaupapa, they still feared me. What a social worker! She did more harm than good. She was always like that. That was her way. She would meddle, interfere with our private lives. She hounded three or four of us guys who were trying to make a go on the outside. Always, she would come to our work place and tell the bosses we were from Kalaupapa. That woman would not let us alone. OK! So I came back, and this is where I will stay.

Inside, we were once prisoners, but now we are free. My freedom is inside, not outside. We have a good life here. There is no crime, no highrise buildings, no pollution. Maybe leprosy has been a mixed blessing. I'm not bitter about catching this sick. No—no bitterness on my part. But I can say one thing. We all came up the hard way!

50

Male, Part-Hawaiian
Blind, Disfigured, Married
Age: 48
34 years at Kalaupapa

FROM DUST TO DUST

Am I disabled? Can't you see me? Sure I'm disabled.
I'm blind too. I had this disease since I was fourteen. That's
when they first sent me here. First to Kalihi Hospital, then
to Kalaupapa--like the rest.

Why are you asking me these questions? We try to hide
from these kinds of questions. It is a discredit to the Health
Department that they let you in. We try to keep away from
people like you, but the Health Department let you in
anyway.

(Further explanation about the purpose of the interview
and research and statement of support from Kalaupapa
patient Council)

The Kalaupapa Patient Council is good now. The
Council is trying to help all of us inside. That's the only
reason I will talk to you. If they said it is OK for you to do
this, to interview us, I will cooperate. You are lucky they let
you in. They won't let just anybody in to ask these kinds of
personal questions. We try to keep our privacy in here.

Let me tell you one thing. We are a flop as a people.
Why? Because the Health Department never gave us a
chance. We don't have a good education. We never had our
share of education for self-improvement. They say we are a
flop because we have leprosy, but it is because of the Health
Department and the Department of Health, Education,
Welfare (HEW). There has been a lack of good education for
patients over the years, and a lack of good spending of the
leprosy money. Now, it is too late, especially for the older
folks, and maybe too late for me too. I say we were denied a
good education right up to 1969.

Do you know they denied me the right to be a blind vendor here at Kalaupapa for the tourists? I wanted to be trained for that kind of blind vendor work by the HooPono Training program, which was paid for by the Department of Health, Education and Welfare (HEW), by the federal government. That was the purpose of the program. I wanted to be self-employed, to try and pay my own way, to seek training. In the future there will be a need for those kinds of persons at Kalaupapa, especially if this place becomes a National Park. Father Damien may be made a Saint, and plenty more tourists will come here. That is an opportunity for some of us to pay our own way and be self-employed. I had looked forward to that so much, but the HooPono said no. They said it wasn't profitable for me to do that kind of work. But actually, I think they are afraid that I and other handicapped patients could do Civil Service jobs, take over the vending work, and maybe even the kitchen work at Kalaupapa. HooPono trains kitchen staff also, and I think the state fears the competition from us patients. They want to protect their jobs--the Civil Service staff and the state bureaucrats. The vendor operation is in the same category as kitchen work, and all of that is supposed to be state Civil Service. It's a matter of job protection.

So I think this place will be a National Park. Why not let us patients work and benefit from the National Park? We have our rights. Why can't some of us benefit from the time we have spent in Kalaupapa? How can a blind man like me be a threat to anyone? But I say we ain't got the right for real education, us handicapped. In 1946, the Randolf-Sheppard Act was amended by the U.S. Congress to protect the rights of handicapped vendors. It was sponsored by the National Federation for the Blind and the HEW. But HooPono and the Health Department still rejected my application to be a blind vendor for tourists. It was a matter of economics, I think. That's why they deny us work rights inside. So, what they do, they use HEW monies against us, because they discriminate against us. They used leprosy as an excuse, but actually it was economic protection. Discrimination. So, those are some of the kinds of problems we have. That of discrimination--economic, political and stigma discrimination.

How did I get this disease? Well, I had eight other relatives in Kalaupapa. Four sisters, my mother and three other relatives. I also have other relatives who had this illness, but they were never discovered. They were never sent here--they escaped.

Me, I came in when I was fourteen. I finished the ninth grade outside. Then, after I was diagnosed as a leprosy person, I had mechanics training in Kalaupapa before I went blind. Now, you might say I am retired. I have a disability pension. Overall, I am one of the lucky ones. My family and neighbors stuck with me. They never rejected me, but I tried to avoid them after I got the illness. So, I will live the rest of my life here. Because of my condition, I don't have too many choices.

How do people treat me on the outside? I think they avoid me. Maybe it is because of my disfigurement. I have had plenty of bad experiences. Most recently I had an embarrassing experience at the Honolulu Lions Club rehabilitation program. I lived in a half-way house, sponsored by HooPono. The teachers did not want to associate with me. Especially one teacher, she was Japanese. I think Japanese are especially scared of leprosy. Also, even though she was a teacher, I think she was ignorant. I was told she quit her job because of me. This happened in 1975. She did not want me in her class. She was afraid I would infect her and the students, even though I was negative. She was told to keep me in her class. She protested to her supervisor, but was told I was medically safe. I could not give her leprosy. So, she resigned rather than have me in her program. All this in the HooPono program for the blind. That is just one of my many experiences with stigma. Truly, our handicap is other people's attitudes toward leprosy, and towards us. It's the stigma of the name leper! It's not bad enough being blind and disfigured. We also have to fight the attitudes of the public. Yes, I think people are prejudiced against me. It shows in the way they act, like I explained to you.

Let me tell you about the worst experience I have had because of this leprosy sickness. It happened just a few years ago, I think in 1976. My in-laws rejected me. The parents of my present wife rejected me, but this also happened with my first wife. Both of them were nonpatients. The parents felt, since I have leprosy and am disfigured, I should not marry a nonpatient. They called me names, called me a leper. In fact, even the nurses told me that. They said, "You have no business marrying outsiders. You should marry your own kind." You see, the public knows about this disease and they are still fearful of it because of the crab hands, scars on my face, and my blindness. I think people still fear leprosy. They put me down and say I should stay inside Kalaupapa. Not go outside, especially not marry outsiders. Even the head nurse at Hale Mohalu said that. What do you think about that? They say we should not be with outside people, with normal folks. Even some of the staff and nurses feel that way. So, I should be put away and stay away.

What is the best thing about being a leprosy patient? I can honestly say there is nothing good about being a patient. Well, maybe if there is anything good, it is that we can duck the public inside here. That is the truth. We have a right to a private life, to a life of our own. This is our home, right here inside Kalaupapa. This is our world. You know, I don't like the kind of questions you ask me. It's the shits. I have been trying to duck these kinds of questions all of my life. But I will answer this for you, and tell you this. We have a right to stay here and have our peace. It's a nuisance for me to answer these questions. Why are people so ignorant and curious about us? It hurts us, these kinds of questions. We are trying to avoid the problems we have had, to try and forget the past.

Anyway, let me tell you something else, while I'm at it. Our patients are dying on the average of three deaths a year. I blame the Department of Health for the deaths of our patients, because we have poor medical care. Why did _____ die last week? From kidney disease! Why didn't they put him on the kidney machine? Why don't we have a kidney machine inside Kalaupapa? Why didn't the doctor diagnose his kidney trouble? Yet he died from kidney problems. The doctor tells me I have no kidney trouble or heart trouble, and they tell other patients that. Yet we die from kidney troubles. It takes years for kidneys to get so bad that they fail. I tell you

54

they neglect us. There is no good care for us. They don't tell us our medical problems.

Another thing, I had problems after surgery with infections. I found they left gauze and sutures within me, and it caused an infection. The doctors always blame leprosy for our medical problems, yet they don't check for other medical problems. I tried to sue the Health Department, but they were found innocent of negligence. There was a statute of limitations on old surgery and they were protected from blame by the Board of Health law. We don't have a law to protect us. That's why I want to discredit the Health Department. They are not as interested in us as they say. As patients, we don't have the health and strength to fight them or fight for our rights. We feel defeated before we start. We are not animals, but they treat us like animals.

Maybe the worst thing about being a leprosy patient at Kalaupapa is the isolation from real life. I tried, but I feel defeated. What can I do? I stick it out and be bored with my life. Also, I don't have much contact with my family anymore. My family never rejected me, but my daughter from my first marriage, well, we lost contact with one another. Maybe she rejected me. You see, people don't want to be connected with leprosy. With my first marriage (I was out in the community then), there was an automatic divorce because of my leprosy. I reactivated, and leprosy was the grounds for divorce--that was the law. After they confined me again, I couldn't get out to see my wife and child. The Health Department would not let me out. Finally, my wife and child kind of forgot about me. So, today I have almost no contact with my daughter. Today she is twenty-six years old and we are like two strangers. My wife never let me see my daughter when she was younger, even after I became negative again. She relocated. In fact, the Health Department helped her avoid me. That social worker, _____, helped my wife divorce me and kept me from my daughter.

Am I bitter? Sure, I have some bitterness. I feel cheated. I don't blame anyone for my disease, but I am bitter about the stigma they put on me. But, it is my fate. Maybe I got leprosy from birth, but I don't blame anyone. Everything rots away, even the body, and my family's body rotted from the leprosy. From dust to dust. We just rotted away earlier than others because of this sickness. We were not intended to last forever. We are all bound to die and rot away from something. But leprosy is the worst. You don't die right away. First you have to face the public and the people around you. It's the slow torture death.

Female, Portuguese
Widowed
Age: 61
42 years at Kalaupapa

I BECAME ONE OF THEM

Yes, I am disabled. My handicap is nerve damage. My fingers are crabbed up, and as you can see, I live in a wheel chair. It never lets up this disease. Nerve damage always goes on, even today after the new medications.

I was nineteen when they first diagnosed this disease. LIke the rest of the patients, they sent me to Kalihi Hospital. All in all, I have been here forty-one or forty-two years. I think I was twenty when they first sent me to this place.

My philosophy of life is simple. It is to smile at people. I smile, they look puzzled, then smile back. It works, you know. I try to be happy, and make other people happy in some small way. I think I have done pretty good considering I have only completed the sixth grade in school. I have had different jobs inside this place. I worked as a dishwasher, waitress, physical therapy aide, and now I am sixty-one years old, and retired.

How did I get in here? Believe it or not, it all started with a little stomachache. My mother took me to a hospital and they gave me a physical examination. Then, I don't know why, they took my tonsils out. I think I looked healthy, but I had those deep red rosy cheeks. They say, that is a sign of leprosy. You know, my face looked flushed and a little puffy. Dr. _____ noticed my red cheeks. He decided to take a snip of my ear lobe and he sent it out to biopsy. This all happened on the operating table while they were taking out my tonsils. When I woke up, I found myself in an isolation ward. They did not tell me why. But I was not in the same room I had before they put me under. It was a very private room, but private! It had only me inside, and when the nurses came in, they were covered from head to toe by white sheets. But for some reason, I still don't quite know why, they released me. I went home. Just like the rest of the patients in the hospital, they sent me home.

Later, my mother became ill, and we had to send her to the hospital. I remained at home, doing housework with my sisters. My throat was still sore from the operation, so I remained home most of the time. But one day, my family went to visit my mother in the hospital. But, they would not let me into my mother's room. The others could see, her, but not me. "Why?" I asked. They did not tell me why. So I went home. A few days later, while I was cleaning house and playing records, a tall, Hawaiian man came to the door. He said, "I got papers here that say you must come with me, go to Kalihi for mai Pake." What? Me? That was the first I found out about it! I had one day to get ready. He came on a Thursday and I had to leave on Friday. I was in shock. I went to our bathroom to look for poison to drink. But I was so shocked and confused, I could not find it! That man who came to the door, they called him the "bounty hunter." He got ten dollars a head for each leprosy person he arrested.

Kalihi Hospital was not too far from where we lived in Honolulu. My mother went with me on the streetcar to another doctor who previously worked at Kalihi. There, they did another snip on me again. They told me I was negative, but that I would still be confined to Kalihi. We could never understand that, and it has never been explained to me. I was negative, yet I was committed anyway. It was terrible.

In the beginning, I used to run away from that place. I would try to get back to my home, especially during periods like Christmas. I wanted to be home so much. But for us lepers, when you ran away, they would put you into isolation-- solitary confinement, like they call it in prisons. Or, you had another choice. You could volunteer to be sent to Kalaupapa. When people were sent to Kalaupapa, we thought it was to die. It was final.

At first, I was afraid of the other leprosy patients. The feeling of fear and sadness exhausts you. One time this lovely lady patient told me, try and cry. Try and cry. I was holding it all in. Later, I did cry and felt better. Before that, other patients approached me and tried to make me feel better, but I was frightened of them. One girl offered me some candy, you know, crack seed. "You want some crack seed?" she asked. "No." I was scared to take it. Here I was confined as a leprosy person, and I was scared I would catch the disease even worse. Also, I kept thinking in my own mind, "I am negative. I am negative." But finally, I accepted my fate. I took some crack seed and ate it. I took, and I became one of them. When the Board of Health saw that I was adjusting and feeling better, they put me to work for nine dollars per month in the laundry. Still, I saved some money.

Terrible things happened in Kalihi. People were so desperate after being sent there. One day somebody committed suicide. We patients gave the Board of Health the name, the Board of Hell. They never got anything done right, even today they don't.

Where do I want to spend the rest of my life? Well, that's an easy question, right here at home in Kalaupapa. I have spent two-thirds of my life here. My roots are here. You can't pull out roots like that. This place is easier for me to live in, due to my condition and all. On the outside, strangers shy away when they learn I am from Kalaupapa. I don't tell strange people I am from Kalaupapa. I let them find out for themselves. Usually there is a guessing game we play. "Where are you from?" they ask. From the neighbor islands. "Oh, what island?" Molokai, I say. "What part of Molokai?" Oh, the country side, I say, or the far side, west end. But we keep getting boxed in. Finally we say we are from Kalaupapa. Usually that ends the conversation.

On the outside, in the old days in Honolulu, they called us lepers. They used to gossip about my family, saying, "Watch out, her daughter is a leper." Funny. The one woman I remember who used to call me a leper, she got the sickness herself. Today, I think people are still prejudiced against us. Especially the Health Department. They are prejudiced just like the rest of the public. For instance, they say we are free to leave Kalaupapa, anytime. Yet we must get permits to have our own family come visit us inside. And we can't bring in our grandchildren. The family can only stay two weeks in the guest houses. Why can't they live in our homes, like family? And if we are not contagious, why do they try and keep out our families? I think they lie to the public. Maybe we are still contagious? Why the difference in the law? I can go out and stay with my children and grandchildren for long periods of time. Yet they can come here only for two weeks, and no children can come in under fourteen. Why?

Nothing will convince me to leave Kalaupapa. Now, I can leave to visit my children whenever I want. But I am resigned to this place as my final home. We all make the best of our lives here. This is it for us. This is the end of our fight. You know how it is. First, you catch the disease. You want to remain home with your parents, and they also love you and want you home. You fight against the isolation. I didn't want to believe my fate. So you fight it, you don't want to accept it. You fight yourself, the disease, the other patients, the Board of Health. Then, finally, you give up, and find yourself. After being sent to Kalaupapa, we find love, we get married, even have children. All inside this place. People on the outside don't figure us as human beings. Maybe they still think we are monsters. But we have our affairs, our lives.

Overall, when I look back over my life, I have been lucky. My family never rejected me. And, I found a wonderful husband. We had a good life together. I am still close to my family, and to my children. You know, my children were born inside, but my family hanai them. So I see my children, and my grandchildren. I am lucky!

I don't take any medication anymore. I stopped taking the medicines years ago, just like many of the other patients. They want us to keep taking the sulfones, and they keep giving us the medication, and we accept it. But when we get home, we just put it into the ice box or the medicine cabinet. Some people have the medicine laying all over their house. It piles up over the years. Only if I reactivate will I take my medicine again. I don't want to develop an immunity to the sulfones, so I refuse to take them now.

No, I am not bitter, but I used to feel anger about my life. But not now. I don't blame anyone for my disease. I don't know how I caught leprosy. No one else in my family had it. So, who can I blame? Inside Kalaupapa is where I should be. I didn't go to church much on the outside. I was lazy. Maybe that is why I caught the disease. But I got my religion inside Kalaupapa.

Male, Part-Hawaiian
Partly Disfigured
Age: 36
31 years at Kalaupapa

MY BIG KALAUPAPA FAMILY

My disease was first diagnosed when I was five years old. It was before sulfone therapy, so I am now partly disabled. My hands and feet are crabbed up and I have some marks on my face. Now I am thirty-six. I have been a leprosy patient for thirty-one years. I have been at Kalaupapa most of the time, but actually I have been in and out of this place. I was declared inactive or negative, and discharged; then reactivated as positive again. It has been going on that way for many years. But for the most part, I have been a patient since I was five.

My father was also sick with leprosy. It's in my family, this disease. When I was diagnosed as a child, my father was waiting for me here at Kalaupapa. You know, my best years, the most happy years of my life, were my early years at Kalaupapa. My memories of home life outside Kalaupapa are not too good. My mother had eight children and my father was away in this place. Life was hard on my family--hard on my mother and brothers and sisters. My family had more children than they knew what to do with. My whole family worked in the taro patch on the windward side of Oahu. All the kids helped my mother. After my father was sent away to Kalaupapa, my mother had three more children by another man. So, there we were, eleven children in the family. After I got the illness, my brothers and sisters were envious of me being sent to Kalaupapa to be with my father. I did not have to work as hard as the rest of my family that stayed behind on Oahu. They had a hard life outside. My life as a leprosy patient was easier.

When I arrived at Kalaupapa, I was the youngest child inside the place. My father was waiting for me when I arrived, along with many of his friends. All the people took me in, and I became like everyone's child. It was really one big family in here, an <u>ohana</u>. I had everything ... so much love! I was spoiled rotten. I even had the nuns taking care of me.

After the war, the sulfone medication came to Kalaupapa. They gave it to me around 1949. After a short while I was declared negative and discharged. I was not happy about that! It actually broke up my life again. Being declared 'cured' forced me to make new adjustments and I was told I would have to leave Kalaupapa. I was around ten years old then, and confused. I had adjusted to Kalaupapa and found much happiness, then I was forced out of the settlement. They sent me back to my mother where life was much harder for me. She was poor and had all those other children. I didn't get nearly as much attention and love as I got at Kalaupapa. I became so unhappy in my mother's home, and each night I prayed for this sickness again. I wanted to get leprosy again very bad. Even though I was young, I did not take my medication when they released me. And I got my wish! One and one-half years after my release, I reactivated. When the doctor found out, he said in a serious tone, you will have to go back to Kalaupapa again. I was so happy. I don't think the Board of Health knew they were making me so happy. I felt I was coming back to my real home. I have been a patient almost continuously since that time. This is my home, and my happiest years were spent here among my big leprosy patient family.

I finished the twelfth grade inside at Hale Mohalu. My main interests have always been drafting and sewing. I am really interested in clothes designing, but I have been working inside Kalaupapa for seventeen years as a kitchen helper. I am really waiting to get my pension from the State. When I am thirty-nine or forty, then I will decide what to do with the rest of my life. I think I am too young to stay inside this place for the rest of my life. I have too much going for me now. I can sew. I can design clothes. I will get my pension and I will get social security disability payments. Then, maybe I can make it on the outside. Of course, this place is still good, but it is not the same as it used to be. It has changed. People are more cold now, and so many people have died. My closest friends have died. Those who raised me, most of them died. But I don't think I will ever leave Kalaupapa completely. Maybe I can make it my part-time home--like a summer home. When I was a kid, there were many patients my age--hundreds of them. But many either went home after 1949, or passed away. I am still the youngest inside Kalaupapa. This place is still good. There is no pressure here--no financial pressure. I have peace of mind inside; it's so quiet. But I don't think I will stay. I'll try and make a go of it outside. I have a lot going for me.

What's the worst thing about getting leprosy? You know, I can't answer that. It never crossed my mind. I don't feel shame or rejection when I am outside. People treat me OK outside this place. There is no prejudice towards me. I don't know, maybe the worst thing was the separation from my real family, but like I said, I was happy here. Since my father was a known leprosy patient, when they found the spots on my right ear, they sent me away real fast. But that made me happy. Maybe the worst thing about the illness is the effect of the medication and the problems caused by the disease itself. I have a loss of feeling in my hands and feet, and that makes it hard to sew and do my designing. Also, I am getting kidney problems and stomach problems--I think from the medication. I still don't take my medication steadily, because of the side effects. When I feel myself reactivating, then I take it again. But like most of the other people in here, I avoid taking my medication regularly. It's the side effects we don't like.

The best thing about Kalaupapa today is that I can save some money. I have easy living. I'm just plain lazy, maybe. But this place is not the same . It is deteriorating; buildings are falling apart. And the people have changed; we are not as close as we once were. But I'm not bitter about my life here or about the disease. I was happy at Kalaupapa, but I'm not as happy as I once was. That's why I leave Kalaupapa often. I go to Honolulu quite a bit.

Male, Japanese
Blind
Age: 62
34 years at Kalaupapa

NO MORE FAMILY TIES

I was a first class carpenter. When I got my flare-up and they found leprosy, they sent me to Kalihi. But I wanted to go to Japan for treatment. I heard treatment was good there, so the Board of Health released me and I went. But in Japan it was no different. In those days, they had the same kind of treatment--chaulmoogra oil. So I came back to Honolulu and was sent to Kalaupapa. I took up my old line of work inside here. I was a carpenter again. But in 1968, I went blind. It was an accident, not related to my illness. The kerosene weed burner blew up and hit me square in the face. That's how I lost my sight completely.

My family is all dead now, except for my twin brother. He lives somewhere in California. Many years ago he told me it was better for his children to break off family ties with me. I was cut off from my family. In the 1950s my brother took his family to California. He did not want them to find out about my disease. So, that's how it is. I have no other family now. This is my only home. It's for good.

Orientals have the most fear of this disease. Like I said, I was cut out of my family. It's like I am a dead duck. When members of my family died, I was never mentioned as a surviving relative in the obituary section of the daily newspaper. It was like I never existed in my family. My family never visited me here. Never. Nobody. So I am a free man. I will go on until that day comes, then pau, finished, I will die. Only my brother is left. So I have no contact whatsoever with family. But I am not angry. I guess I understand. In the beginning everybody was scared of this leprosy. You can't expect them to come here all the time; but for me, they never came, ever. But I can't blame anybody. How can I blame anyone? I don't know how I got it.

No other people in my family got it. No friends got it. Me, I'm just a hard-luck man, I guess.

When I die, I don't want my family to come here. Don't notify anybody. Just forget it. I just want to be buried and be done with it. That's all.

Male, Japanese
Partly Disabled, Divorced
Age: 60
41 years at Kalaupapa

THIS PLACE IS HEAVEN

I was nineteen and a clerk in the plantation office. I noticed I had some numbness in my calf. I had first contact with leprosy when I was sixteen; a friend of ours had the sickness, so I was afraid I might get it. Before I went to the doctor I asked about the illness. A friend's father told me to test myself. They said to hold a lighted match to myself. If you don't feel the burn, you got the Molokai sickness. Well, I lit a match and did it, and I felt nothing. That's when I knew for sure I had the leprosy sickness.

I was sent to Kalihi and then here. The worst thing about my being sent here was what happened to my family. The feelings in Japanese families are very strong about leprosy. Orientals are more prejudice and fearful of the disease than other races. But everyone was frightened of it in those days, and my getting the Molokai sickness put my parents in a tough spot. For instance, after it became known I came down with leprosy, few visitors came to our home. Worst of all, my parents lost their jobs, my mother as a maid to the plantation manager and my father as a yard man. And my family worried about my younger sisters, if they could get married or not. Before, it was thought this disease ran in families, that it was inherited. Even some of the staff members who worked with us were ashamed to tell others they did leprosy work. One nurse at Kalihi Hospital was shunned by her friends for working with us. But I was lucky. My family did not shun me, and my sisters found husbands. Today, they always ask me to visit them on Maui, and I do. So maybe I don't feel as isolated as some of the other folks.

I don't blame anyone for this disease, and I don't feel bitter. It was God who sent me to Kalaupapa; it was His work. I found religion and my faith inside Kalaupapa. Today

I am a Catholic. Before, I had started to drift away from the church. On Maui as a Catholic, we were told not to associate with Protestants, and I thought that was too strict. But being a Catholic in Kalaupapa is better. So I am happy. I feel now is the happiest time of my life. Nothing will make me live outside Kalaupapa. This place is heaven, I would say.

Female, Japanese
Disfigured, Blind
70 years of Age
40 years at Kalaupapa

AKERAMERU

I had disgraced my family and my husband with this disease. The Orientals--the Japanese and Chinese--feel much shame about leprosy. They try to hide leprosy because of the disgrace it brings to the family. It goes against your family forever. The new ones born after you, the ones already dead, and your ancestors are disgraced. We believe in ancestry, and leprosy spoils your ancestry. For the Japanese, leprosy sickness is recorded in your family history in the Koseke-tohon. Each family's history was written in it. Also the Yakuba--a central place for family records in the neighborhood. We had it in Hawaii too. After a disgrace like leprosy, other families would avoid your family and maybe not marry your children. It could not be a secret because it was recorded inside the family history. That is why some people with the disease would just disappear, go away. They were not kept in the house--no matter if you poor or rich. They just would go away out of the house. This way might not record in the Koseke. If you die you just die. Family history has no record then of leprosy.

My family had many problems after I got the disease. To help them, I keep away from my family members. I don't go out and I don't mix. They have a family business and I don't want to hurt them in any way. So I keep away. I go out of Kalaupapa one time a year. I see my daughter at Hale Mohalu only. I never go to the family home. They would be disgraced.

All of us have had problems with this disease. People mistreat us because of the disease, they do not show respect to us--even some of the staff. The head nurse especially at Hale Mohalu. You know, we have feelings, we can understand. But one time when I was at Hale, the head nurse

69

treated me like a monkey. She would not even say hello to me when a tour of nurses came through the ward where I was staying. She was showing me to other nurses. She displayed me, me a real leprosy patient! I think professional staff like that look down on us. But we are not dirty, we are not monkeys. But, leprosy is leprosy. It will take many years to wipe out the prejudice and fear people have of us. It will take a long time before they figure out we are just people. But I think little by little, things are improving. For instance, on the television news, now they talk nice about leprosy patients.

Today, I think about my illness, my life, and I feel very sad for my family. I feel shame, and I feel bitterness also; but I accept it. In Japanese, we say, "akerameru" (I accept my fate).

Let me say something more, I don't want to be sent from Kalaupapa to some old age home. This is my home. I don't want to be mingled, mixed with non-leprosy people. These are my people. I am old, blind, crippled, and helpless. Let me stay here forever.

The things I tell you, this was all thirty years ago, maybe more. As far as I know, that's how it was.

Male, Part-Hawaiian
Widowed, Blind, Disabled
Age: 80
65 years at Kalaupapa

THAT WILD GERM, BUCKING LIKE A WILD HORSE

The disease caught me when I was seventeen, in 1914. The tall Hawaiian health officer, the one they called the bounty hunter, came to get me at school. Nobody knew I had the sickness at home. We didn't suspect anything was wrong with me. I was only seventeen years old; but somebody reported me at school, and that man came. They took me away fast. From Puna, to Hilo, and to Kalihi Hospital in Honolulu. That all happened a long time ago. I don't think about it much anymore; it's too late to do anything about it. It all happened to me a long time ago. When I think about it, though, I still hate the trouble I had with this disease. Yes, maybe I am very bitter about my life. I don't blame anyone for the leprosy problems I have, because I didn't know I had contact with any leprosy persons before they sent me away from my family. But I am bitter. I wish I was dead three years before I was born. But, what shall be shall be. I think I am just an unfortunate human being. I used to feel the leprosy germs inside me bucking like a wild horse--that wild germ!

The worst problem I have had was the separation of my body from my blood and flesh on the outside, from my family. Most of my family is gone now, but I did get married inside, and something good came from that. I have children, and twelve grandchildren and great-grandchildren. So I am lucky that way. I don't leave Kalaupapa much, except to see my children and my moopunas. I go when I am in top shape, when I feel good. That is about once every three years. My children were raised hanai style by my family. So I was lucky there too. I never was rejected by my family.

Because of my condition, I usually stay inside Kalaupapa. I will stay here until I go into the belly of our ground.

71

There is no use me trying to make a life on the outside. When I do go out, most of my time is spent at Hale Mohalu. My family always comes to visit me there. I don't like to go outside Hale, not even to my children's home. I think sometimes, people still fear folks from Kalaupapa. That's why we keep to ourselves. It's more comfortable to be among blood and flesh, and friends. I don't like to be with strangers. I know that in the old days people did not like this disease. They had fear of being contaminated. Also, we looked like apes. Today, maybe people are not as afraid as before, but maybe some are still curious.

So I will stay at Kalaupapa. They try and do their best for us. But there is no direct cure for us. We got caught in the old days, and we suffered. That's why I am blind and disfigured. Those new drugs can't help me now. I think those fellows who drank plenty of okolehau (alcohol) were helped by their drinking. They made home brew in the old days. Some of those fellows were not as bad off as me. I never drank the stuff, never touched it. Maybe that's why I had the bad effects from the leprosy. But my old gang is out now, make, dead. So maybe some angels were good to me ... or maybe I was good to the angels. That's why I'm still alive.

Well, because of God's great love--here I am. When I visit with my grandchildren, they make me feel like a diamond in the blue sky. That's good because I am one of the oldest people in the settlement. I been here since 1914. And I will stay here until they put me into the belly of our ground.

Female, Filipino
Married, Able-bodied
Age: 41
8 years at Kalaupapa

LOVE COULD NOT OVERCOME FEAR

I got the disease when I was thirty-three years old. I came from the Philippines and married a local Filipino man in Honolulu. I had a good job working for the military in Honolulu. But one day, my eyes became red and I lost some weight. I had red blotches on my hand. My husband sent me to the doctor at Tripler Hospital, and he told me it was the leprosy. He did a biopsy and it came out positive. Four days later he called my hous∙ and said I should stay home--not go to work. That was in 1968 or 1969. He told me someone from the Health Department would come to my home and explain my disease to me.

Well, I was married and my husband became very worried about this sickness. The Health Department nurse said we should not worry, that they could cure me pretty fast. She said I must go to Hale Mohalu for medicine and stay inside there until I got better. I stayed there over one year. But my husband got funny feelings toward me after that. He was cold, and his family never came to see me. I think they were shamed by my leprosy sickness. I was becoming lonely inside the hospital. So I asked my husband to stay with me. The hospital allowed spouses to stay with patients one night a week. But my husband said no, he did not like to be with me. He did not want to eat with me, and he did not want to sleep with me. So we drifted apart. Later we got a divorce. I felt terrible because I felt like I was being thrown away by my family.

I came to Kalaupapa voluntarily. I met my new husband inside Hale Mohalu. He understood how I felt, and he was kind to me. He was a permanent resident of Kalaupapa and he asked me to marry him, and come and live in Kalaupapa. I agreed and that's how I arrived at this place. But, first I got my negative status at Hale Mohalu. I was declared negative. Still, even though I could have left Hale Mohalu, I decided to come to Kalaupapa with my new husband. I am not sorry. I have a good life here and I help take care of my husband.

I don't have many problems, not like the other patients inside here. I have no scars on me. Those new medicines helped my condition. But still, Kalaupapa is my home, even though I don't feel prejudice against me on the outside. The only prejudice I have felt was from my ex-husband and his family. That was enough for me.

Male, Japanese
Divorced, Partly Disabled
Age: 55
42 years at Kalaupapa

I PAID MY OWN WAY TO CARVILLE

(Interview conducted at the U.S. Public Health Service Leprosarium, at Carville, Louisiana)

I was thirteen when I got this disease--one of the young ones. I am like the rest of our Kalaupapa people, except that I was the first Kalaupapa patient to come to Carville for treatment in 1970. I paid my own way. I had heard about Carville, read about it, and I needed surgery. Other patients who required corrective surgery usually were sent to St. Francis or Queens Hospital in Honolulu, then they went back to Kalaupapa. I wanted something better. My arches were broken down (drop-foot), so I had trouble walking. I had seen so many of those patients get operations in Honolulu, especially for foot problems; but after they returned to Kalaupapa, they would break down again. They would wear only tennis shoes because the orthopedically-designed leather shoes are not available for our people. I tried to make my own shoe padding for my broken arches, but it was futile. We did not have good specialized help for these kinds of problems. Actually, there are no leprosy specialists in Honolulu and no good orthopedic surgeons who know about leprosy patient problems. So, I decided something must be done. I decided to pay my own way to Carville.

I got my first good medical treatment after I arrived at Carville. The Chief of Surgery told me I should never have gotten in such bad condition. I arrived in Carville in a wheel chair because I could not walk. He said my medical condition had been neglected in Hawaii; I had not gotten the proper treatment. After my surgery, I wrote to other patients at Kalaupapa and told them how good the medical care was at Carville. Soon, others came. They paid their own way just like I did. Later, around 1973, the Department of Health started to pay our way here for special surgery; but before that they always said they did not have enough money to send us here.

If you go to Kalaupapa, you notice people wear Keds tennis shoes and rubber boots. Those tennis shoes are not good. They are not like orthopedically-designed shoes because Keds stretch when you walk. Within two months after foot surgery at St. Francis or Queens, our people's feet would break down again. That is why people with "drop foot" continue to have foot problems in Hawaii. There are no prescription shoes designed and manufactured by an orthopedic shoe man. Finally, sometime last year, the Hawaii State Health Department sent a fellow out here for a two-week study course on how to make orthopedic sandals. Now they have a sandal maker in Hawaii, but still no specialized shoes.

I am a believer in the Carville system of medical care for leprosy patients. I have learned much about my disease at this place. That's why I stay here; I get better here. At Kalaupapa, I feel my condition deteriorating. Let me tell you what kind of a staff they have here in Carville. They have the kind of professional people that are unavailable to our Kalaupapa people. First, they have a specialized foot doctor He supervised the making of real orthopedic shoes for us. They have a physical therapist and a vocational rehabilitation staff to serve us. They have a psychiatric staff, dermatologists, full-time social workers, and full-time doctors for us Kalaupapa patients. You know, that Kalaupapa patients have not had a full-time doctor for many years. One doctor visits Kalaupapa two times a week. He spends about twelve hours a week there, and we have 128 patients. Another thing, they have a dialysis machine here. There is no kidney machine at Kalaupapa; yet many of our people have kidney problems, and they die from kidney failure. They also have education specialists for us. We have classes at Carville. We even have a recreation specialist. I try to convince as many of our people to come here as possible. Today, there are five of our people here. In Hawaii, we don't have health professionals in charge of the leprosy program. At Carville, there are real professionals in charge.

I know about my disease because it seems like my whole life has been wrapped up with my illness. I got the disease when I was only thirteen. I was removed from my family and sent to Kalaupapa. I really don't know what life is like on the outside since I have been institutionalized since I was very young. They caught me in school. The principal of the school was suspicious of me due to a swelling on my neck. Also I had hard red lumps on my cheeks. So they sent me to the doctor. They made the diagnosis in Hilo, then I was sent to Honolulu.

My home has been Kalaupapa since those early days. Now I spend more time at Carville since there is more hope here. I think I have adjusted pretty well, but when I was in my early twenties, I became desperate to be part of the outside world. I felt life was passing me by. For instance, I wanted to try something--anything that might help me. That's how desperate I was. Well, I read an article in Collier's Magazine that horse toxin was being experimented with as a possible cure for leprosy. I immediately volunteered for horse toxin injections. Up to that time, I was in pretty good shape. But after the injections were given me, I had terrible reactions. That was around 1944-1945. After I volunteered for that experiment I blew up. I had terrible reactions, I blew wide open. I was very sick. I had swelling, sores all over my body, high fevers. But because I was so desperate, I tried anything to get rid of this disease. But instead, I went downhill. That was the turning point of my physical condition. It made me worse. Some of the other patients used as guinea pigs also suffered from those experiments. But like me, they would try anything to get out of Kalaupapa. I still consider Kalaupapa my home, and I will return back there when my physical condition improves. But for now, I will stay at Carville because of the good treatment that is available to me.

I really don't go out that much. Oh, in Louisiana I go to Baton Rouge sometimes, and to New Orleans. There are no problems. But sometimes people stare at my hands or the marks on my face. Maybe I am overly sensitive. No, I don't have too many problems on the outside today. Still, I will never live with my family. I don't have problems with my family, they accept me, yet I feel protective toward my family. I don't want to hurt them. Should I expose myself to others when I am with them, it might embarrass them.

What is needed is more public education about Hansen's disease--leprosy. The public should be educated about this illness. They should know what doctors are doing to help patients at Carville and that the disease is not highly communicable. Maybe national television should focus on the public education problem. That is the only way to reach the people and get the true information across to them.

Male, Part-Hawaiian
Blind, Disabled, Married
70 years of Age
57 years at Kalaupapa and Hale Mohalu

THE STATE HAS PROVIDED:
I AM GRATEFUL TO OUR BENEFACTORS (AT LEAHI)

I have many stories, many. But I will tell you the main part about my life and you can see if that is what you want to hear. But first, you tell the people not to be concerned about us leprosy people. Don't be concerned about us at Kalaupapa or at Hale Mohalu at Leahi. We are happy. The State has been good to lepers. Tell the people the State has provided. They are our benefactors, and we should show appreciation for what the State has done for us. I am grateful to our benefactors . Without the State, I would be dead. Not all of the patients think that way. Some are hotheads, trouble-makers. Yet I think the Board of Health is doing all they can to alleviate our suffering. The Director of Health has love and compassion for sick people, and he is trying all he can to help us. So tell them not to be too concerned. We are like people anyplace else. We love, marry, drink, murder, commit suicide, fight. We have all the human drama. We are everything you are on the outside. Just like that --life is life.

They caught me in school. I guess you heard that one before. I was in elementary school in Honolulu. I made it all the way to the sixth grade, and then suddenly it was all over. One day out of the blue, the principal came to my classroom. He said something to my teacher. Together they pulled me out of class and took me to the principal's office. From there he told me to call my mother. I did, and he then took the phone from me and spoke to her. I really did not understand all that was going on, but I could hear my mother crying on the other end of the telephone. I started to cry too, because she was crying. I was only thirteen years old. The principal told my mother to immediately take me to the Kalihi Receiving Station for lepers because I had the mai Pake. I guess he knew the signs of mai Pake. My face and hands had been swollen for some time before that. But we were poor, so my family didn't take me to the doctor when the swelling started.

My father came to take me home from school; but instead of taking me to the Kalihi Receiving Station immediately like the principal said they should, my parents took me home. There we all cried. The whole family cried, including my father. The next day my father took me downtown and bought me a new suit. It was my first suit of clothes--they were so nice; I looked good. I had never had clothes like that before because we were poor. Also, where would I have worn those kinds of clothes? But I wore a tie and everything ... new shoes. My father bought me a complete new outfit. So I wore that suit of clothes to the Kalihi Receiving Station. Even though we were poor, my father said he wanted me to be dressed nicely when I was taken to Kalihi to be declared a leper. They took my picture for the official record of the Board of Health wearing that new suit of clothes. When the picture was taken, my father broke down again and cried. So, I became a leper.

It was hard for all of us, being taken away from our parents like that. But in Kalihi I learned a lot. I became a Catholic, and I still am a Catholic to this day. I became an altar boy and learned about the love of God. I began to learn about the importance of suffering for our Lord. God has eased my suffering, and I know when I die and leave my body here, then there will be no more leprosy for me in the kingdom of God. Satan and Hate has never bothered me, and I even have love for the man who later in my life seduced the girl I was to marry--the man who took my wife away from me. It's hard to love Jesus Christ.

Well, many things have happened to me, so many things. There are many stories. But let me tell you how I was first sent to Kalaupapa. During my time, minors were not sent to Kalaupapa except if parents requested their children to be sent there, or for punishment. You see, leprosy may run in families. Some families wanted their children to be cared for by relatives already at Kalaupapa. Or in many instances, parents of young children were already confined at Kalaupapa. But in my case it was different. I had no relatives at

Kalaupapa and my family in Honolulu did not want me to be sent further from them. There were no requests made to send me to Kalaupapa. I was sent there for punishment over the strong objections of my mother and father. It happened this way.

After being declared a leper at thirteen, I lived at the Kalihi Receiving Station for four years. I began to adjust to my new life. My family would come and visit me, but the Board of Health was very strict. You could not touch your parents or other non-patients. So that is how it was. We could talk to one another only by a separation of space, ten to twelve feet of space was always between us. On my side of the space, in the visiting room, was a small table and a chair. On my parent's side, a small bench to sit on. We were separated further by a strong wire mesh, stretching from floor to ceiling. It was on the visitor's side. In this way, there could be no touching between relatives and confined patients. There would be no passing of objects to one another. So you see, the disease was considered very contagious in those days, and they took great care to separate us. We were thought to be a threat to society. One day, after my parents' visit, when they arrived home they found a bright yellow sign on their gate in the front yard. It was put there by the Board of Health. It read "QUARANTINE NOTICE. This house has a communicable Disease-- LEPROSY, and is subject to Fumigation." That was the Law. From then on, all those who passed our home knew there was leprosy in the family.

Well, I was becoming accustomed to my fate at Kalihi and I think my parents were too. I had become very religious and also was active in the Boy Scouts. As a matter of fact, I was a Senior patrol leader of my troop. My troop had a real good drill team, and I was proud of that fact. Every morning we would go out and march and do our drills. It was good exercise and I enjoyed it. But then we had a conflict. Some of the other patients were jealous of my troop and so they started their own drill team. Then we had two drill teams. Us, the official Boy Scout drill team, and the other drill team made up of adults who were not boy scouts. But we were the official drill team, the Boy Scouts and members of the Honolulu Boy Scout Council. So that's how the conflict started. The adults and the administrator of the Kalihi Receiving Station wanted my troop to drill with the adults, but I refused. We were the official drill team, members of the Boy Scouts of America. We were organized first, and we drilled and became good long before the new adult drill team was formed. The other team was composed of just leprosy patients, just a group of adults headed up by a patient. I think they envied the prestige I got as a Senior Patrol Leader, since we had uniforms and all the official insignias, even though we were just leprosy patient kids. Well, the adult patient leader of the new team wanted to be a leader too, and he wanted my official team within his own team. I think he was a man of some importance before he became a patient. He seemed to have influence over the other patients. Outside, he may have been a man of some prestige. But once you become a patient, that's it, you become a patient. A leper. I think he wanted something more inside, and I did too.

So I was sent to Kalaupapa as punishment. I was in the way of the adult patient drill team leader since I refused to cooperate with his new drill team. I had no reason to cooperate. I had my own troop and drill team. So I was punished and railroaded to Kalaupapa for my beliefs. In fact, the Honolulu Times ran a headline stating, "Young Boy Railroaded to Kalaupapa." The administrators of the Receiving Station supported the adults. I spent six months in Kalaupapa before my parents managed to get my release. My mother got an attorney and went to court. She received a writ of habeas corpus looking into the matter of illegally sending me away to Kalaupapa as a minor. But it took her six months before she could set me free. All the while I remained at Kalaupapa, the nuns took care of me. Then the President of Health (he was called the President then, not the Director of Health as they are now) came to Kalaupapa. Dr. Trotter was his name, and this building at Leahi, where some of us patients stay, bears his name. He made a special trip to tell me I would be free, free to go back to Kalihi Receiving Station. So that's how it was I was summoned to his house. Of course I could not go in because I was a patient. I stood outside his gate and he told me I was free. That's how I went back to Honolulu. I left Kalaupapa wearing my Boy Scout uniform with all of my insignias. On my sleeve I had the Boy Scouts of America patch. It was a kind of triumph for me.

When I arrived in Honolulu, my mother and sisters were there to greet me. Of course we could not touch. Then I learned my father had died. Only my mother and sisters were left. Yet it was one of the happiest moments in my life, to get back to Honolulu. My mother couldn't stop crying, nor my sisters. I cried too, but this time I knew why I cried. I finally knew the meaning of being a leprosy person. Like I said, outside you could be anything, belong to anything, be a person of prestige. But once you were declared a leper, you became a leper. Everything else didn't matter, you could be sent to Kalaupapa for any little thing, not only leprosy.

In 1927 when I was nineteen, my name came up for return to Kalaupapa. This time not as a punishment, but as an "incurable." I told my mother not to struggle. I was becoming a man and I had to take it. My return to Kalaupapa was not to a foreign place. After all, I had spent six months there earlier, and there was a particular girl I wanted to see again. It was the girl I was to marry at Kalaupapa in 1930. She was a non-patient, the daughter of confined leprosy patients. She was one of the few who were allowed to live in Kalaupapa as a child without the disease. Actually, they had assumed she had the disease from birth since she had a birthmark on her face. Maybe she was the only non-infected child who was allowed to live with her parents in Kalaupapa. They kept her there thinking the birthmark was a sign of leprosy or might turn into leprosy in the future. But she never caught the disease. She remained at Kalaupapa until she left me for another man, a non-patient Board of Health worker who seduced her into committing adultery. I never remarried, but remained at Kalaupapa alone. Although leprosy was grounds for divorce and she asked me for a divorce, I would not grant it. You see, I am a Catholic, and we took the vow "until death do us part." But I still love her, even though she had children by the other man. That is not an easy thing to take.

As far as I am concerned, life goes on. I love God and love my neighbor. Because of my love of God, I survive, regardless of my afflictions. I will carry on until I am called back to my God. And there, after death, there will be no more pain, no leprosy, no bad memories. I hold no bitterness or grudges. I can do nothing else, but take up our Lord's cross and follow Him, and with His love, I survived.

A VIEW FROM THE OUTSIDE

A Family's Accounting

A letter translated from the Hawaiian,
by Mrs. Ruby Johnson, Associate Professor
of Hawaiian, UHM.

Dear Mrs. Johnson,

This story is about my grandmother, about how her son
got leprosy. She made every effort to keep the matter from
the Board of Health, so that they would not take him away.
So, the family hid him. Inside their house. He went from
island to island on steamships. On one of these trips, the
Board of Health was waiting for him on the dock. They, the
Board of Health, knew about him, and caught him. They
packed him off to Kalaupapa. From then on, mother and son
were separated. This happened in the 1920s, before I was
born. The information is contained in her letter written in
1947 after her son's death. It was for the record, for our
family genealogy.

He wrote his mother from Kalaupapa telling her he was
ill. He knew he was dying. He asked her to come see him at
Kalaupapa, before his death. But, as he grew worse and lost
strength, the Board of Health sent him to Honolulu--I think
to Hale Mohalu. But by the time my grandmother reached
him, he was ready to die. Too late. After all those years of
separation she finally lost him. This is the story about her
last contact with her son, maybe her only contact with him
after so many years of separation. This is her story about her
trip to Kalaupapa to bury him.

(The translation from Hawaiian and the telling in English.)

Written on Monday, <u>March 1, 1948</u>: My son contracted
leprosy in the 1920s while working on ships. He avoided the
Board of Health for several years until they caught him. He
was the oldest son.

85

<u>March 1, 1947</u>: I received a letter from my son at Kalaupapa asking me to travel quickly to see him because he was put to bed in the hospital, in October.

My thoughts were so disturbed and fearful at this news which arrived. I decided to ask for help from my other children. First I asked one daughter for help, then my son. Finally, I asked my other son to help my daughter get me a room and passage on the plane for Kalaupapa, I also needed a paper from the Board of Health giving me permission to visit my dying son. All this happened a few days before the weekend. I wanted to leave on a Saturday morning.

Finally, I got an answer from my daughter. She called from Oahu to tell me I would not be going to Kalaupapa because my son had already been brought to a hospital in Honolulu on Thursday. So, my trip was shortened. I then insisted to my daughter that she please get me a ticket for the airplane on Saturday, if she could. My daughter agreed that she would let me know on Saturday morning and for me to wait for her answer by telegraph. I agreed. I waited for my daughter's answer. Her reply came at <u>10:30</u> a.m. <u>March 6 Saturday</u> morning telling me that for this day there was no room. But, she was successful in obtaining a reservation for me on Sunday morning, at 8:30 a.m. I agreed.

I told my son that I would be away in Honolulu to see his older brother. When my son heard the news, he decided to go also, thus to see his older brother. He asked me if the two of us should go to the office in _____ to ask for another space on the airplane. When we arrived at the office, the agent told us, there was room only for one. It was my son, then, who was to fly first to Honolulu, on the very last plane on Saturday. I would go the next day, Sunday.

<u>Sunday, March 7, 1948</u>: My things were ready. Also my grandchildren. We all left home at 7:30 a.m. for our flight and to check for my ticket paid for in Honolulu. When we arrived at the airplane office, they began right away to check about the ticket. Soon their checking was over. Our tickets were brought out. At 8:30 the plane left for Honolulu. When we emerged from the plane at Honolulu, all of my

86

children and their wives and husbands had arrived. Happy this meeting of the mother and all of the children.

I praised God for this trip.

In the late afternoon all of us went to see my weak son. I went to see him all of the time, every day, except on the stormy days.

The second week, he couldn't come outside, and we were allowed to go inside.

So we continued to do this until the morning of <u>Tuesday</u>. On <u>March 23, 1947</u> at 9:45 a.m., he left this life. With great sorrow for my child!

True is the word of God. Dust returns to dust, and the spirit with God.

I praise the kindness and love of God.

My last visitation to him was quickly taken care of. At 10:30 a.m. I saw him. When all of our visitations to him were over, his body was taken to be burned to ashes.

His ashes were ready on Thursday. We were notified that a plane would be flying to Kalaupapa to carry freight and other things. Then this little box of ashes would be sent on that plane. However, this was not the will of God.

Thursday. My daughter knew about the urn and other matters. She phoned the hospital office and told them that my mother wants to fly to Kalaupapa to see the conclusion of her son's burial. The Hospital Head said, your mother can't go at this time because the visiting place at Kalaupapa is too full. Maybe wait till next week.

So, my daughter took proper care of everything. These things were all left up to the head of the hospital.

Here was our plan:--

(Daughter speaking):

1. We fly to Kalaupapa. I, my mother and two of my sisters.

2. To please take care of the funeral arrangements for Sunday, at 2 p.m.

3. To please inform Lawrence Judd, administrator of Kalaupapa.

4. To please get us a special plane, a charter.

5. To please inform them that we must return to Honolulu at 3 p.m., after the burial, after "Nalo" . . . he is out of sight.

The head told us it would be possible for me to set all of these things in order. I must get a special permit to take my box of ashes, the ashes of my son. He told me, to please come on Saturday morning to get the box of ashes, the urn, and the permit for burial at Kalaupapa.

My spirit praised God that we did not have to struggle with these tasks.

March 28, Sunday: We left home and arrived at Andrew's airfield base on Oahu. The pilot was already waiting for us with our tickets. There were four of us. It cost $75 round trip for us all.

After 9:15 we left for Kalaupapa. I holding the urn. When we began to fly we were in the mist flying like smoke, through which Moloka'i was seen. But when we came closer, this mist opened up until we saw one half of Moloka'i and as we came near the shore, then we saw Kalaupapa.

Fine the steering of our pilot, a Japanese. Fine how he made his decisions on flying the plane.

Our pilot navigated until the landing field, then Lawrence Judd came to the plane, with some other friends of our family. A little rain began.

Lawrence Judd took the four of us on his car to the house of _____. Here we were welcomed with warm affection.

A meal was prepared quickly for us, and we gave the urn to Mrs. _____ to be carried by her to the church.

On the table were all delicious things. Kalua pig, raw fish (aku), crab, ele'ele seaweed, chicken, cake, and we ate until enough.

Great was our appreciation for the kindness of the friends of Kalaupapa. When the meal was over, we decided to go to see the home of my son. It was furnished nicely with everything, but he never lived long enough to enjoy these things. Everything was beautiful. What sorrow. When we returned to go to the church. The raindrops fell from the sky.

When we were led inside, oh, how beautiful everything with which it was decorated. On the table was arranged the urn of my beloved son. Orchid leis on his urn, and his table was adorned with white crown flowers.

It had been done so properly.

It had been taken care of with such reverence, and now only the grave, was the last thing.

By the grave, the rain cleared up for the very last rites, for my "wreath," my dead child. Afterward, we went straight to our plane.

Lawrence Judd was there and he gave us a certificate for our leaving a member in Kalaupapa. This paper certified we had no more family inside Kalaupapa.

We thanked everyone. We had been welcomed with love.

We thanked the loving God by whom all things are made right.

Unforgettable love. I am going someday again, so that I might once more see the grave of my son.

This is I, _____
the Mother writing (for our family records)
(March 1, 1948)

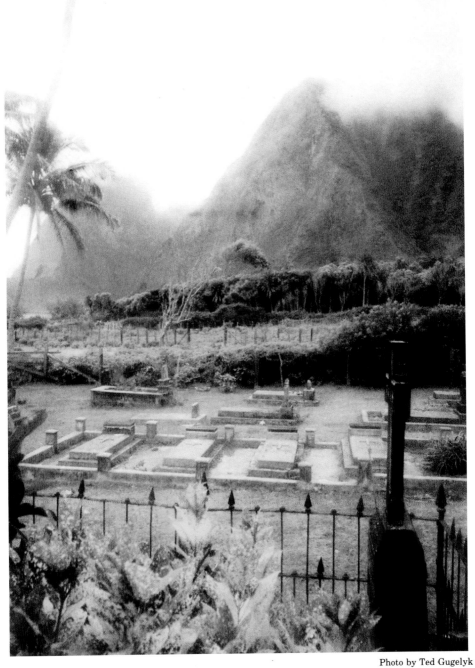

Photo taken from Father Damien's church, Kalawao. Damien's grave is in the foreground. His remains have been taken to Belgium.

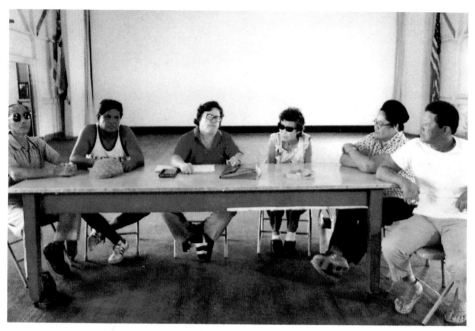

Kalaupapa Patients' Council

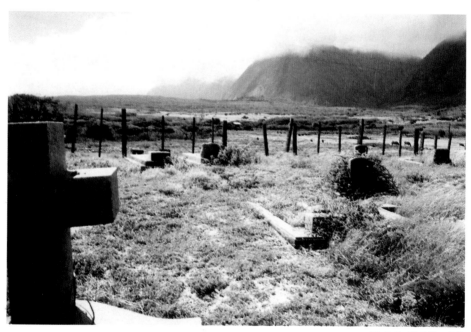

View to the east of Kalaupapa Settlement showing graves and Kauhako Crater

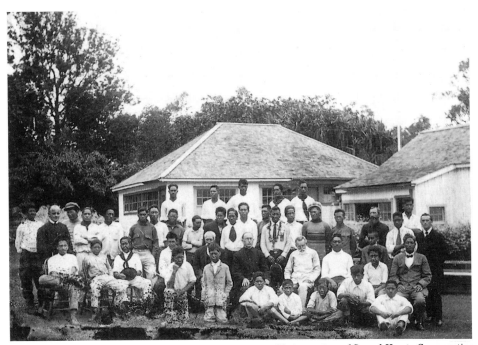

Sacred Hearts Brothers and the boys of Kalawao. Brother Joseph Dutton is seated center right in white. (circa: late 1920s)

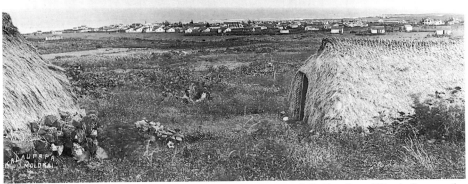

Early Hawaiian grass huts alongside the newly constructed Kalaupapa community, after the move from Kalawao (circa: between 1884 and 1904)

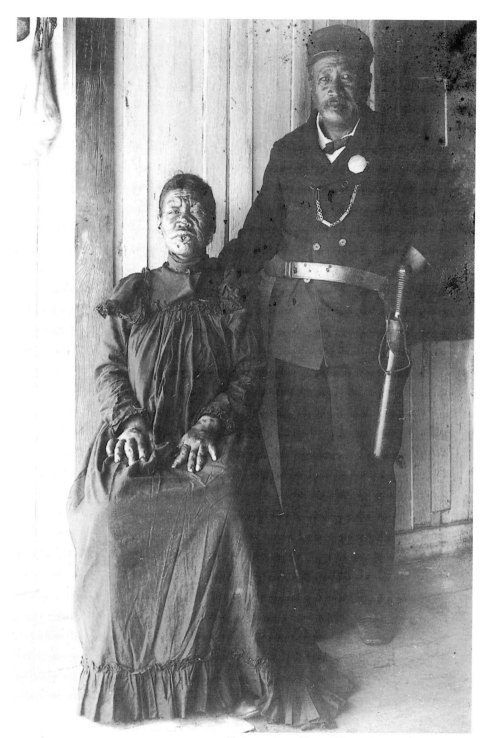

Law enforcement officer (a helper or kokua*) and his wife, a patient at Kalaupapa (circa: 1910–1920)*

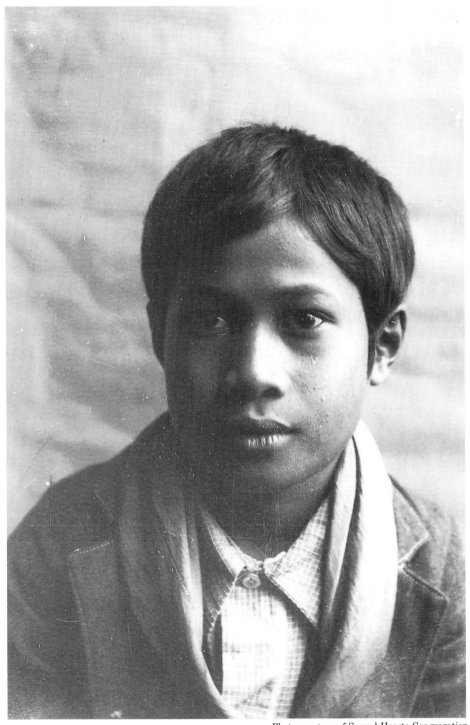

A young boy with leprosy. Photo taken before disfigurement, but after confinement at Kalaupapa. (Date unknown)

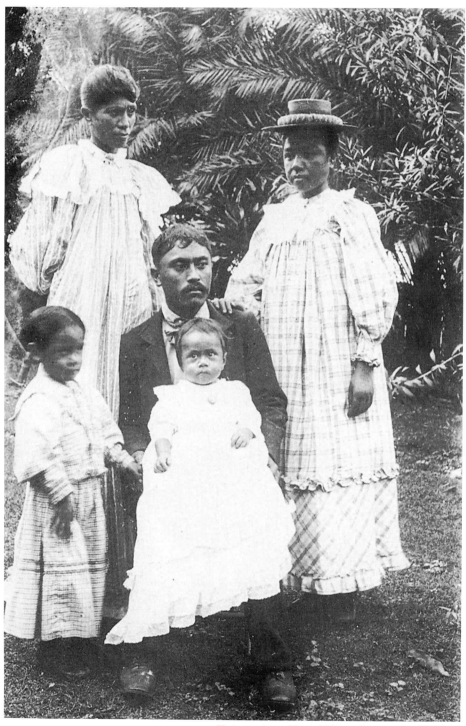

A family in confinement at Kalaupapa (date unknown)

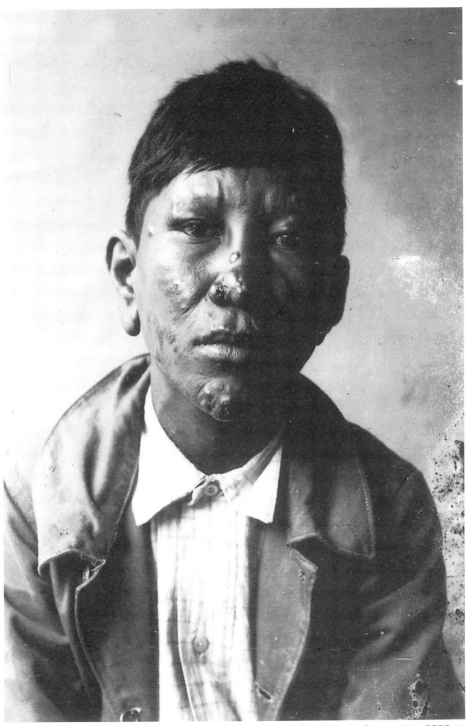

Photo courtesy of Sacred Hearts Congregation (SSCC-44)

Progressive disfigurement caused by leprosy (date unknown)

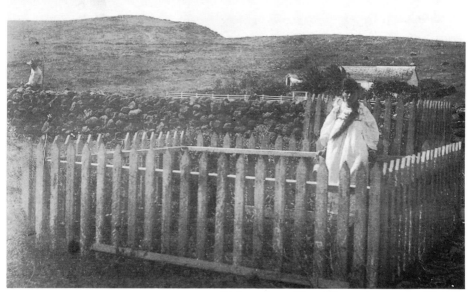

Graveyard plot at Kalawao (date unknown)

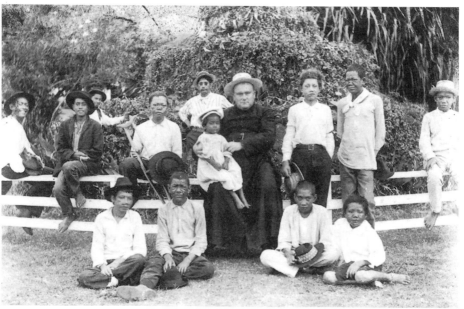

Father Ulrich Taube with leprosy patient children at Kalawao (circa: early 1900s)

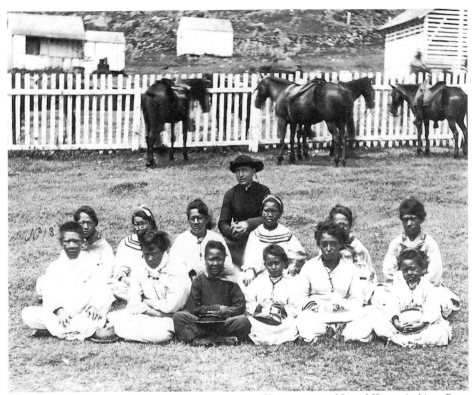

A still-healthy Father Damien with the Girls' Choir, at Kalawao (circa: late 1870s)

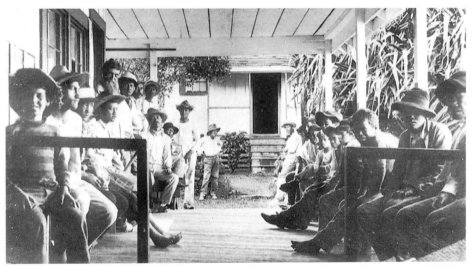

Brother Joseph Dutton (with beard) at Baldwin Home for Boys, Kalawao (circa: early 1900s)

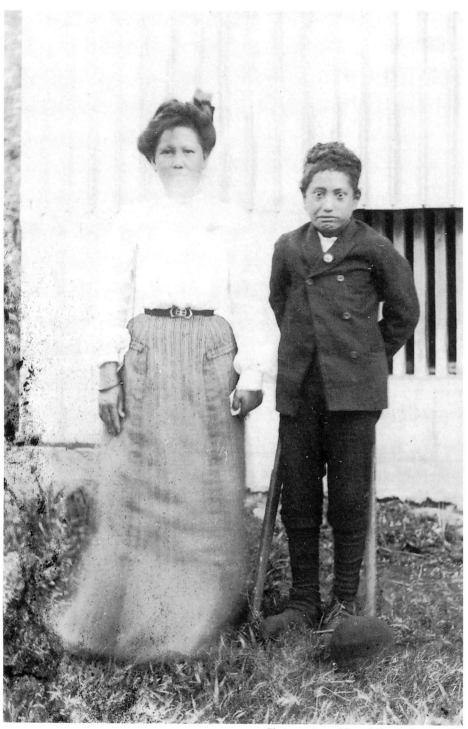

A patient poses with his mother at Kalaupapa. (Date unknown)

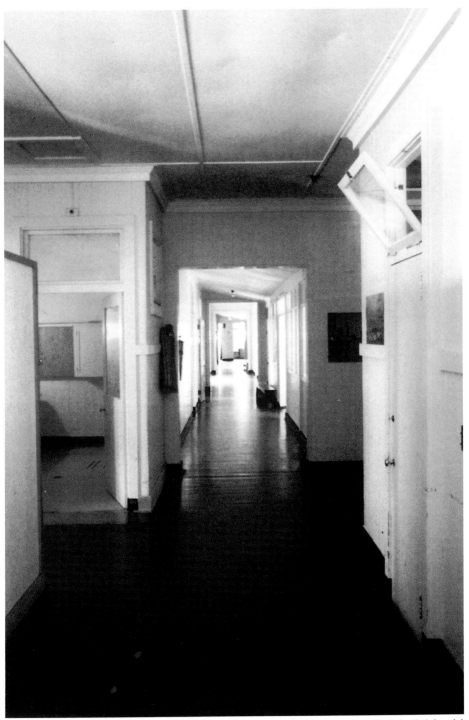

Old hospital at Kalaupapa—view of main corridor

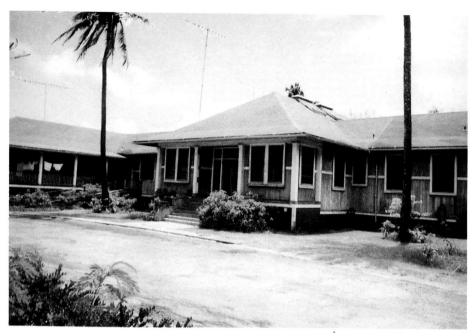

Photo by Ted Gugelyk

Old Hospital at Kalaupapa built in 1932, provides daily nursing care for 7–12 patients. (New hospital completed 1979)

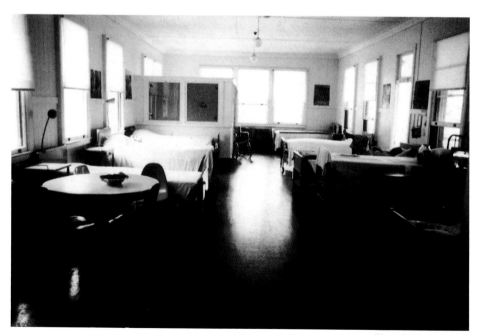

Photo by Ted Gugelyk

Old hospital—men's ward.

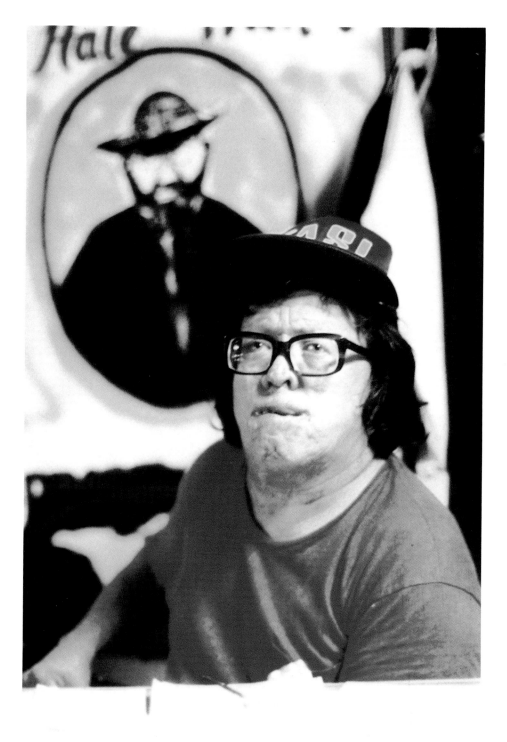

Photo by Ted Gugelyk

Bernard Punikaia, Chairman, Kalaupapa Patients' Council

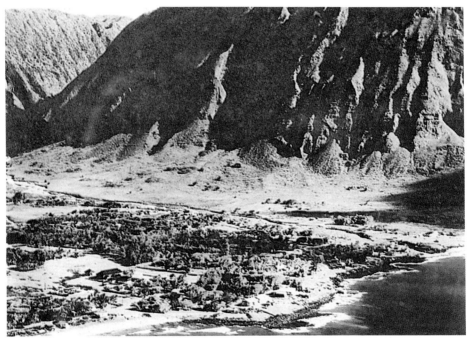

View of Kalaupapa taken during the 1940s

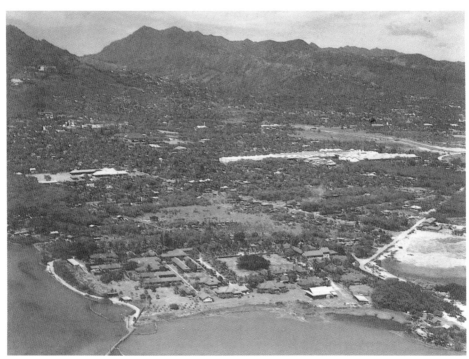

The old Kalihi Receiving Station, Honolulu (circa: 1939)

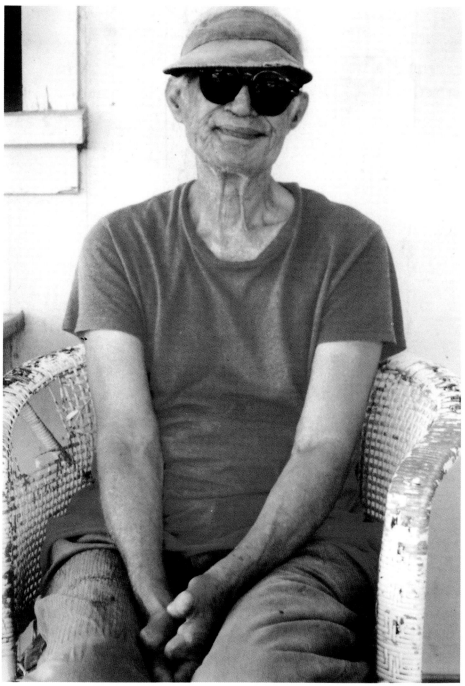

A senior resident, age 80. Sixty-three years at Kalaupapa.

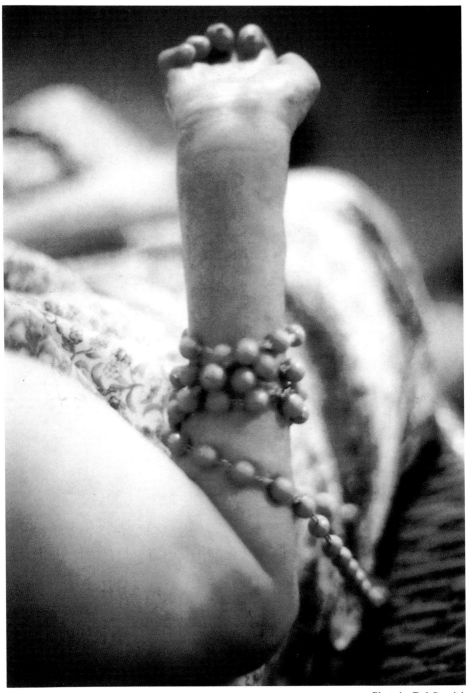

Bone absorption—one of the effects of the disease.

Part-Hawaiian Male
Blind
43 years old
31 years in confinement

THE LONG ROAD--

from Papakolea to Kalaupapa,
to a University Degree

I am forty-three years old and it has been a long road for me. But things have been getting much better in my life. I just graduated from the University in May 1978. I have a Bachelor's Degree in Liberal Studies. My interest is Hawaiiana. I want to become more familiar with my cultural heritage, and maybe teach others about my culture. But it has been a long road. There was a lot in between my being declared a leper and where I am today, and where I want to go with my life. But I feel good. Things have gotten much better for me. I am climbing up from the dependence of being a leprosy patient. I have always hated dependence, having others make decisions for me. Finally, my life is leading to more independence. It's a kind of growing up.

My story started right here in Honolulu. In Papakolea, the Hawaiian Homestead community on the side of Punchbowl above Honolulu. My parents were taro farmers in Laie. Our whole family worked the taro patches, me included. But when I was twelve, my family suspected I was coming down with the sick. Growing up, my family and I, we were already familiar with the word leprosy, mai Pake. I had three family members already at Kalaupapa. My two brothers and one sister. So our family was familiar with the sickness. It caught our family. When I showed the signs, I too had to see Dr. Chun-Hoon.

That doctor had diagnosed the rest of my family members, and then he diagnosed me. We had no choice in going to see him. I was reported, turned in to the Board of Health by my sister's ex-husband. It was a family matter, and he wanted to get even with my family. You see, after my sister was sent away to Kalaupapa, my mother hanai her children ... my mother raised her grandchildren. But my sister's ex-husband wanted the children. My mother wouldn't give them up. So, he turned me in as a kind of revenge.

Anyway, I went for my mandatory check-up on a Friday. That is the day the Board of Health said I should go. Within one hour of my check-up, I was told I would be committed to Kalihi receiving station. Also my father. My dad had a cut, an infection on his leg. He got it working in the taro patch. The doctor assumed immediately that it was the leprosy. Later, they found out it was not. So my father was released, but I stayed. That is the kind of power they had over our lives.

On October 3, 1947, I was sent to Kalaupapa, because I had family there. The Board of Health sent anybody. Adults, children, anybody. If you were not responding to treatment, away you went. The same week I went, many other patients were also being transferred from Kalihi to Kalaupapa. A few years before that, patients were either sent on a steamer, or sometimes, on cattle barges. Yes, they were sometimes sent as steerage. But we were lucky. I had a one-way trip by air to Kalaupapa. Lawrence Judd was the administrator of the settlement at that time. He helped start the air service.

So there I was, a young boy from Papakolea, going to Kalaupapa. You know, it really didn't dawn on me what was happening. I was not excited, I was not frightened. My parents had accepted it. I was just going to be with my brothers and sister. But, today I have some thoughts about what was going through my head at that time. You see, my parents raised their own taro. They ground their own poi, in the old Hawaiian way. It was all work, work, work at home. And I was ashamed of being Hawaiian. I was not proud of being Hawaiian. Many people were ashamed of being Hawaiian then. I am just another dumb Hawaiian working in the taro patch. So, I was happy to go, to get away. Also, I wanted to be like my brother. I thought my brother was lucky. He received presents from my family. He got a new bike. I never got those things. I thought, boy, maybe I can ride his new bike at Kalaupapa. I had no profound thoughts about my leaving. It was just like one adventure. A little boy, thinking maybe he too would get gifts.

But when I arrived at Kalaupapa it was a surprise. I didn't know what to expect. Kalaupapa was a real community, a small sleeping town. Everything was well kept, and I thought, there are so many cowboys and cowgirls here. You see, patients walked around the town with handkerchiefs around their necks. I thought they looked like cowboys in the movies. But they had had tracheotomies. So they wore the handkerchiefs around their necks to cover up the holes in their throats. It kept them breathing. But I thought, what a town, filled with cowboys and cowgirls!

I wasn't frightened by what I learned and saw. I never saw hideous cases of leprosy, but they were there. I wasn't scared. I just began to live another life, and I was closer to my brothers and sisters. My brother though, had medical problems already. He had one "flare up" when I arrived, a reaction to leprosy. He was red, and all swollen, with a fever. Still, I wasn't scared. Also, I didn't feel any shame or stigma, as you say. I knew on the outside, leprosy was not something you talk about. But here, on the inside, there were so many of us, so leprosy was just a way of life, in a community of lepers. It was like one big family.

Like kids anywhere, we had to go to school. I entered the eighth grade. But school was backward at Kalaupapa. Our books were old. They were the same books I had used in the fourth grade in Honolulu. They were discards, sent to Kalaupapa. The teacher was a patient, and the school was only three hours per day. So I began to get bored. There was no challenge. But we couldn't play hookey. Where could you go? And if they caught you, look out, you would get punished--the doctor would spank the dickens out of you. Plus my parents would hear of it, and get angry also. No, there was no place to hide. But I was bored with school. So I got sassy. The teacher told me that if I did not shape up they would expel me. That was too humiliating. To get expelled from school at Kalaupapa. Everyone would have heard of it, especially my parents. But I really did not learn anything in

93

school, but I stayed, and my behavior improved. I think school was just to keep us out of the way. They didn't know what else to do with the little kids.

But we did work around the settlement. They gave us clean up jobs, like that. Also we had our monthly "progress." This was a check with the doctor regarding our condition. Dr. Norman Sloan was the Kalaupapa doctor at that time. They would check our leprosy condition, to see if the sulfone drugs were helping us kids. For some reason these drugs never helped me. Dr. Sloan would also check little things, like our fingernails. If they were not clean, he would put us across his knee and spank us. The kids worried about those "progress" days. One kid put a book on his behind, so that his spanking would not be too bad. But of course Dr. Sloan found out, and gave it to him that much worse.

Kalaupapa kids also had what we called, the "lobster club." That was the nose treatment. They would stick applicators up your nose. They were soaked with some kind of medicine . . . to break open the mucus and tissues in your nose. It hurt. Those applicators remained way up our noses for 15 or 20 minutes. We looked like lobsters walking around that way.

Oh, they had a lot of rules for us kids. Like we had to always wear shoes. Little things like that. We were at the mercy of the Board of Health so much, even for little things. The Board had complete power over our lives. Even punishment for little infractions of the rules. Me, I thought, my parents are my God, they have the right to punish me. Not the Board of Health.

Another thing I remember about my childhood at Kalaupapa, was how the people looked forward to being released. They had to go through what the Board of Health called snips. That is, they had to have six snips taken over a period of one year. They would take skin scrapings in search for active leprosy bacillus. Also a biopsy and nose scraping. The whole process took twelve months. It was heartbreaking. Sometimes people would be negative on five of them, then fail the last one. So many patients broke down and cried,

94

even the adults. Failure meant one more year at Kalaupapa. For some, it meant a lifetime.

Little by little, I got worse--different parts of my body started to go. I lost sensation gradually. My ears. My hands. Feet. Little by little. I had so many medical problems. They put me on the sulfones. But they didn't work for me. I really don't know why. The disease never got any better for me. I kept going, from bad to worse.

I finished the eighth grade about 1949. That was the year about the big outcry, concerning the proposed closing of Kalaupapa. They closed Kalihi Hospital, opened up Hale Mohalu, and were anticipating moving the people out of Kalaupapa to Hale Mohalu. But the patients refused to go. They did not want to be moved again. That was so much their history, movement against their will. A lifetime of it. First from their homes, then to Kalihi, then to Kalaupapa. As far as the people were concerned, Kalaupapa was the last move. So, they remained at Kalaupapa.

But us kids, they moved anyway. We had to go to Hale Mohalu for school. I didn't want to go. I chose to remain behind at Kalaupapa, since I got used to the place as my home. But my family urged I return to Honolulu to Hale Mohalu. There I finished school, finished up to high school. I graduated from the Hale Mohalu high school in 1952.

After that, I began to have other problems--eye problems. By 1964, I started to go blind. By January 1965, I was blind.

To me, going blind was especially traumatic. I resisted public acknowledgement of my blindness. I did not let the staff know how bad my eyesight really was. I was blind for a few months before the staff found out. I could still function within my room and in the hallways of Hale Mohalu, but it was hard. I would try to avoid people. When they fed us, I would eat in my room. I would eat alone in my room, and try to feed myself. But I had no sensation in my hands, so the forks would fall from my fingers. I resorted to eating from the plate, with the use of my hands. That was the only way I could eat. But nobody saw that. Since I didn't want people to see me stumbling around, I would fake things, to hide my blindness. I would say I was tired, or pretend I was distracted, or sleeping. I did many things just to avoid people.

I hated to be classified with the blind. I was still young, yet the blind were always off by themselves . . . a separate people among leprosy patients. They had their separate little community, a separate circle of blind folks, left to themselves by other patients. It was like a final place for me. A place I couldn't leave from. It meant I would be more dependent. Losing my independence, I hated it!

After a few months the staff found out. Officially, I had to join the community of blind leprosy patients. My parents found out. They were very sad, and cried. I had to move to the blind side of the hospital. I fully intended to shut myself into my room and never come out. My room became my world. That way, I wouldn't get hurt. I had my radio, my weights, my talking books. I closed myself off completely. I left the world before my friends left me. That was how I intended to protect myself.

But as things happen, I was helped by a very sympathetic and understanding patient, a girl. She helped me come out. She forced me to re-enter the world, without pity for myself. I think my turning point came when I offered to push an old man, without legs, in his wheelchair. He was ashamed, to have one blind person pushing him. What a pair, he thought. But I said, never worry. Just tell me which way, straight, right, left, whatever. So, that's what we did. We became a pair--a blind man pushing a legless man. That brought me out more than ever. I found out I could make friends again and leave the separate world of the blind. Also it separated friendships, like the separation of the wheat from the chaff. People offered to help me, to help me help myself. Others rejected me.

I would practice walking with my cane late at night. I would leave the ward and walk around the many acres of grounds at Hale Mohalu by myself--sometimes for hours.

Occasionally I would get lost, not be able to find my way back. There was no one to help me, at 3 or 4 a.m. That's what I wanted, to be on my own. Of course, I had to fight off panic, lost in my dark, in the dark. But I kept a cool head, and would try to retrace my steps. Where did I go wrong? Did I go right, when I should of gone left? But I always found my way back, sometimes at dawn, just as the other patients were waking. That gave me confidence to be on my own, while they were sleeping, safe in their beds.

But still, I had many frustrations, and it was an uphill fight. I lacked privacy. Many blind folks do. I was still dependent. Officially, I was classified as blind, and officially that meant I was helpless. Nurses would enter my room at any time, even when I was dressing or undressing. No privacy. So again, in time, I started to feel nobody gave a damn, because I was blind. I began to drink heavily. To escape. To feel frustrated, and feel sorry for myself. What I really needed was a way out for myself. A way out of the small world I was locked into. My world was Hale Mohalu Hospital, the blind ward. I tried to break free, but it was so hard.

By 1968 my frustrations continued to build up. I was drinking very heavily. Then the Board of Health started talking again about moving us. They wanted to move us out of Hale Mohalu, to Leahi, or Kaneohe. There we were, about to be moved again. That made me very angry. Decisions were being made for us, without our taking part in those discussions. As I have said, I wanted to be independent, and that Board of Health planning emphasized how dependent we all were. So, I took part in some community discussions. and served on some committees, I began to get involved again. That brought me out into the world once more.

Then I met another girl, a non-patient. She was a practical nurse at one of the hospitals. We fell in love, and it made me feel good. To think an outside person could take an interest in me! My life started to look up again. That inspired me to try for more freedom. To break away from an environment of people making decisions for me.

In 1970, Hoopono, the Vocational Rehabilitation Center of Hawaii, became interested in me. They encouraged me. I wrote a small story for a blind magazine, and won a prize. That gave me confidence to try and do more. So, I moved out of the blind ward, away from the dependence. I took up training with Hoopono. I received mobility training from a special instructor and I learned to walk around more.

Also, Voc. Rehab. suggested I try university work. I had taken tests which suggested I was potential college material. It was in 1972 that I entered the University of Hawaii.

What a fantastic experience! I was frightened, yes, but excited! A new life was opening up for me. I learned there were many blind students like myself. I felt accepted by them, and other students. So, really, that was the beginning of my new life. I was starting to have confidence. I continued with the University. I even moved into the dormitory.

Money has always been a problem. Especially with dormitory housing. The Health Department has not helped me with my education. I had applied for monies from the Health Department Lani-Booth Fund, a fund for patient rehabilitation and research. They have a fund of $250,000. I applied for $80 for a new tape recorder to record my lectures. But I was rejected. However, the Kalaupapa Lions Club helped me. Also, the Vocational Rehabilitation Department, of the State, came to my assistance and supported me in my studies. I have also received some Social Security Supplementary income. That is how I got through school.

You know, at first I felt so self-conscious in the dormitory, especially in the cafeteria. I know the young kids would stare at me. They were not too sensitive. I would drop my eating utensils. It was frustrating, and they didn't know what to make of me, a blind leprosy student. But I made friends slowly. Now I am a familiar figure on campus. Most of the time I feel comfortable. People stop and ask me about leprosy. I graduated with a B.A. in May, 1978. Next, I will get my professional diploma for teaching, my fifth certificate. I want to teach. Maybe also do some counseling.

There are alternatives for me now. My life has changed. When I first went to the U.H. I had three things on my mind. I wanted to learn to speak Hawaiian. I wanted to write and learn to sing well. But now I have other interests. Maybe I am still self-conscious about my looks, but I want to look ahead and overcome my appearance hangups. I want independence. A profession. I am headed towards some dream. Before I lost my sight, I remember pictures of the East Coast, Vermont, Connecticut--those places. I want to go there. I want to feel what it is like living and studying in another part of the world. My dream. To get a Master's Degree at an East Coast university. Maybe people will accept me there, as they have here. I never want to go back to the muck and mire of the blind ward!

Male
Part-Hawaiian
Partly Disfigured
48 years of age
37 years in Kalaupapa

LEADERSHIP

Bernard Punikaia
The Chairman of the Kalaupapa Patients' Council

<u>My Early Life</u>

I am a Kalihi boy, born in Honolulu, on Republican Street. Actually, I grew up in the downtown section of Honolulu, by River Street and around Aala Park. I went to school in that area. My school was called Robello School, but it's not there anymore. It was located where the Honolulu Community College now stands. I remember those days, at Robello, when I was just a kid. One of my most vivid memories was at the age of six. The railroad trains were operating in those days, and I remember walking to school and stopping on the railroad trestle to watch the old Dole pineapple train ramble by.

My family was an Ohana, an extended family, big like most Hawaiian families are. But in our home, there were only five of us under one roof. My mother and stepfather, my brother and sister and myself. During those days, very little out of the ordinary happened in my life. I was born a Hapahaole (Hawaiian-Caucasian), raised by my mother, went to school, and I was no different than the kids of that period. We would play baseball, and on weekends especially during the summer, go to Aala Park. The city would turn on the fire hydrants on hot days and we would play in the cold gushing water. Just like kids anywhere, that's how we were. I was happy and growing, until the day I was taken away.

How did it happen? There was no leprosy in our family. I don't know how I got it, or that I had it. One ordinary day, the visiting school nurse noticed a red spot on my cheek. Immediately arrangements were made for me to see Dr. "Kuli" Wayson, a leprosy specialist. "Kuli" means deaf in Hawaiian--he was hard of hearing so they called him the deaf doctor. But he wasn't deaf to the signs of leprosy. My mother took me to see him at the Board of Health Clinic on Vineyard Street. I was taken into the examination room, stripped naked, and placed on a little revolving platform. I was spun around slowly, to be observed from all angles by various doctors present in that room. It was a bare room. I was only six years old, and alone with them. They were strangers, and I felt very alone, frightened and inhibited. I still remember the first question they asked me when I was on the examination stand. Dr. Wayson asked me if I was attending school. I said yes, but he didn't hear me. He was deaf. So he said in a loud voice, "Speak up, speak up, boy." It really frightened me because he was speaking in such a loud manner.

After the examination my mother was told to take me back home, but we were ordered to return to the clinic in one week. The plan was to officially order my confinement in the following week. I was to be taken to Kalihi Receiving Station. The one week at home, after the examination, was to help my family and I become accustomed to the idea that I had leprosy and that I was to be put away. I can still recall reaching home, after the examination. I was changing into my play clothes. I heard my mother crying and explaining to a neighbor I had the separating sickness, that I would be put into Kalihi. Then for the first time I began to wonder what kind of a place they were sending me to, since my mother was so upset about me going there. So, I became worried too. What were they going to do to me? Although I was only a six-year-old child, I knew they would separate me from my family. But I didn't know it was to be a permanent separation, and neither did my mother. She was told the standard thing, told to the families of all newly diagnosed patients. That is, I would be released in two or three months and returned home. We were told the two or three months' separation was to be an observation period.

You know, I was never considered a "cry baby," so I didn't show too much emotion during that week. When we returned to the clinic, I remember a big Hawaiian man whose job it was to deliver patients to Kalihi Receiving Station. I learned later some called him the "bounty hunter." He sat outside the doctor's office and watched us enter. My mother was extremely upset, very upset that day. It was impossible for her to accept my enforced confinement that day. She was so upset that she kept crying, because she knew I would be taken away from her and put away. Seeing her agony, the authorities said she could have a few more days with me, at home. As yet, we were not ready for the separation, for the parting. So we turned in relief from the doctor's office, and walked out into the hallway. Our relief was shortlived. There sat the big Hawaiian man. He asked us, "Where are you going?" My mother explained to him the doctor's decision to give us a few more days together at home. But the big man said "No!" He stated I must go with him now. If not, he would call the police to forcibly remove me from my home and take me to the Receiving Station. My mother could not refuse his demand. It's hard for me to tell you these things. The memories rush back after the years. It is so painful. My mother just broke down. At that point I was placed in an official Board of Health car, with my mother at my side, in the back seat. We were driven away, directly to Kalihi Receiving Station.

When we arrived, we drove through the big gates into the open compound. We were greeted by many patients who were already confined. They crowded around the car, curious as to who the newcomer might be. I was introduced to the head nurse. I stepped out of the car, but my mother remained within. I noticed there were many children there, but none so young as I. At six years of age, my admission to Kalihi made me the youngest child confined at the Receiving Station. So the patients crowded around, young and old, curious who the newcomer was. That's how it was. We drove through the gate and suddenly I found myself inside. The nurse instructed one of the children to escort me around the buildings, to give me the tour, so to speak. Then my mother and I had one last embrace. She grabbed me and hugged me. I still remember her tears. She didn't want to let me go. The car door began to close, and they pulled us apart. They shut the door, and the car slowly moved away. I stood along the roadside as they drove her off. Then I was alone. And so it began, February 15, 1937.

I had no fear of the people, not the young or the old. Of course, some had the signs of advanced leprosy. Puffy, swollen faces, scars, some were ulcerated. But I wasn't frightened of anyone. I mingled freely with the patients, and ate with the patient children. I had no fear. Because of that, the older children began to respect me, because I was not afraid of them. As you know, some other newly admitted patients refused to associate with the patients, thinking they would catch the disease even worse. Some newly confined patients felt their diagnosis was a mistake, that they didn't belong there, so they too kept to themselves and didn't socialize or eat with the other patients. But not me. In fact, I gained a reputation for bravery. When a patient died, and many did at the receiving station, they were kept over night in the church chapel. On those evenings, when someone died, the older boys wanted to bunk up with me in my room. They figured I was the bravest of them all, and not afraid of ghosts. I was eight years old then.

There were five years spent at Kalihi. But in the beginning, it was very difficult. But people adjust to any kind of new environment, and I did too. As a young boy, I was very extroverted. I was not shy, but always outspoken. Sometimes, that got me into difficulty, because I would speak my mind about different matters. I guess that part of my personality was formed very early. Yet, no matter how good a front I put up during the day, there were tears every night, for my family. I missed them. I looked forward to my mother's visits each Sunday.

What I tell you are only a few of the highlights--there is so much I could say, so much I have not told, about those years. But the events I remember most relate to my separation from my family, the loneliness, especially at night, crying myself to sleep. Also, I remember getting experimented on. I remember the chaulmoogra oil injections, extremely painful. The women fainted, and the men trembled. And of course, I remember especially December 7, 1941.

103

It is ironic, but the Japanese attack upon Pearl Harbor was responsible for sending me to Kalaupapa. By December, 1941, I was quite ill. By then, leprosy had really took hold of me. But that Sunday morning, I was in the hospital yard, and we saw the airplanes come down. They were flying low over Kalihi. Some dove down from the sky and dropped bombs a few miles away on Pearl Harbor. We could see the black smoke and hear the explosions. Everyone crowded into the church for protection. The children were told to pray. But not me. With a few friends, I remained outside to watch the action. I climbed up into a large hau tree to get a better view. I almost got shot by a Japanese plane straffing the neighborhood. The plane was very low, just above tree top. I could see the pilot's face looking down at us, smiling. His bullets made a double line, starting about 150 feet from my tree, thumping and kicking up dirt on to the fish pond beyond. At that point, we all realized this was for real, it was war. Everyone else rushed for the chapel, but not I. It was in no way the safest place to be. I remained in my hau tree, high in its branches, hidden in the leaves. I remember so vividly the planes passing directly overhead. I have so many memories of that place where I was first confined. Even the memories of such a historic event.

It was that event in history which was responsible for us children being shipped to Kalaupapa. Honolulu was declared a war zone, and for us kids, I guess the Board of Health considered Honolulu to be a hazard to our health. Of course, they considered us to be a hazard to society too. But for our protection, and maybe the protection of the citizens of Honolulu, we were told we would be sent directly to Kalaupapa. The decision was made quickly. Some children pleaded with the nurses. At that time, Kalaupapa had a dreaded reputation. It was a place where people were sent to die. It was a place without hope, a final solution, a final place of isolation from which there was no return. Children were normally not sent there, unless they had relatives confined within Kalaupapa. Only the advanced adult cases were sent there. But it was the Japanese attack upon Pearl Harbor which changed the Board of Health policy and thus resulted in my final banishment to that place we all feared. We feared it because we had friends who were sent there.

Only a few returned, maybe for sterilization operations at Kalihi Hospital. But when they returned for the operation, they desperately wished to get back to Honolulu if only for a few days. They had changed so much. Physically they came back disfigured, in the advanced stages of leprosy. All those things we knew and we feared what we thought was to be our final banishment. So that's how it happened.

I was sent to Kalaupapa on May 15, 1942. May 15, 1979 will be my thirty-seventh anniversary there. Thirty-seven years ago I was banished from society and family. My mother couldn't visit me each Sunday anymore. We were sent away from Honolulu Harbor on the ship Hawaii. There were forty-two of us on the ship, almost all children. It was a dreaded day, and I remember it with so many mixed thoughts. One thing, I remember the Kalihi medical staff speculating I wouldn't last six months at Kalaupapa. Because of my advancing illness, they expected me to die there. I was in such poor health. I was weak, had high fevers and chills, ulcers appeared first on my ears then spread over my body. There was no medicine to stop the illness. The ulcers festered. My whole body hurt. I was miserable.

As we were leaving for Honolulu Harbor, again we said our last alohas to our friends who remained behind at Kalihi. What was especially sad was that some sick children's families did not come to say goodbye. It happened that way in families. There was still love between them, but in some families, life began to go on in separate directions. Gradually visits by parents diminished. One Sunday they would not show up, or maybe not the next either. Mothers had other children to take care of, and new children were born in the family. Separate lives began to be lived. So on that day of departure, because of the "Hookaawale" ... the separating or pulling apart of families, some children did not have their mothers or fathers to say goodbye to. Actually, because of the loss of contact, parents did not know their children were being banished on that day. For some children, the final alohas were to fellow patients left behind at Kalihi.

The Kalaupapa memories? Again, there are so many, so much I could say. In a few words, my sickness was very serious. I didn't begin to improve physically until I took the sulfone therapy, starting in 1946 through 1948. My early days at Kalaupapa was mostly a matter of suffering. They are not cheerful memories, not typical childlike memories of baseball, fishing, horseback riding, hunting, none of those things which were available to the healthier patients on that beautiful peninsula. It was a serious sickness I had. I was literally covered with raw ulcers, my hands, feet, face, and I became so hypersensitive to touch--especially on my ulcerated areas. Even the changing of dressings caused extreme pain. There was so much pain that a nun, knowing how painful it was for me, suggested I pray to God asking Him to take away some of my agony. Of course, in some of the advanced stages of leprosy, there is a loss of sensation and pain is diminished. But I did not reach that stage.

The turning point in my life was in 1948. I was seventeen. Sulfones improved my condition. Over the next ten years life began to improve. The ulcers disappeared and I could work and be active. I started then to get involved in sports--baseball, hunting, horseback riding. We had different sports leagues and organized competition within the settlement. Kalaupapa was a viable community then. In those days there were around 450 patient residents. And so, I worked as a patient worker under the State for twenty years. I retired on a State pension in 1970. Also, I finished high school by taking the General Educational Development Test, at Carville, Louisiana. I went to Carville in 1973 for corrective surgery--and while there I completed my high school education.

Life has changed drastically for me, maybe not all by design. After my health improved, I became more involved in community activities in Kalaupapa, and I have always been interested in education and improving myself. I joined the Lions Club and in the early 1950's I became very active in the Democratic Party of Hawaii. I have always been extroverted, and I have always liked politics and discussion. In the early 1950's, then, I became Precinct Chairman for the Democratic Party. I became involved with Maui County politics. I developed working relationships with Elmer Cravalho, now Mayor of Maui County, David Trask, current president of the

Hawaii Government Employees Association; George Fukuoka, Circuit Court Judge on Maui, and many other politicians. So my interest in things political is not new. I paid my dues in Democratic Party work and have been Precinct Chairman for fourteen years. Also, these were exciting times for the Territory of Hawaii. The Democratic Party was building and unifying. The objective was Statehood. I knew Governor Burns long before he was elected to the U.S. Congress as the Delegate from Hawaii. I have always been interested in community work, in politics. In 1968 I represented Kalaupapa as a patient representative to the Citizens' Committee on Leprosy, chaired by Dr. Tom Hitch. I have had many community involvements. I was President of the Lions Club from 1961 to 1962. I became Chairman of the Kalaupapa Patients' Council in 1968. Before that time it was dormant, not active. I think I helped bring it back to life as a viable and active representative of patients' interests. I served as Chairman until 1972. Then I left for Carville, but I remained a member of the Council. Then I returned to Kalaupapa again in 1974 and was reelected Chairman in 1977, 1978 and in 1979. We changed the Constitution of the Council. Now we hold elections each year, rather than every two years. What angers me is that after my most recent reelection in 1979 the charge was made by Governor George Ariyoshi and George Yuen, Director of the Department of Health that I was an outsider, an agitator; it was implied that the Council did not represent the community on the matter of Hale Mohalu and other issues. That is wrong. The Council does represent the community as a whole, and furthermore, 54 percent of the Kalaupapa people vote in the elections.

My Political Activism

I have been Chairman of the Kalaupapa Patients Council for altogether six years. Although I have been elected unanimously by the patients at Kalaupapa, it's a lonely position, being the designated spokesman for the Kalaupapa community and Hale Mohalu. I am concerned both about the future of Kalaupapa and the future of Hale Mohalu, especially the forced move of patients from Hale Mohalu to Leahi. I have always been active in community affairs at Kalaupapa, always been outspoken, but now things are different. People know me within the State and even the

107

Mainland because of newspaper and magazine stories about the leprosy patient struggle here in Honolulu. Also stories have appeared in Time & Newsweek.

I see my place as fighting for our rights. I feel I would not ever, never, give up . . . just throw in the towel! But it is lonely. Many times I feel I am banging my head against a stone wall. I wonder if it is worth it. Even more so when the people whose rights you are defending do not seem to be as interested in their rights. Some take the attitude, "Oh, what the hell, you know, what's the use?" They give up so easily.

Why it is so, is very difficult to define, but somehow some of our people are apathetic about some of the most important issues affecting their lives. But I think this is prevalent not only in our community of Kalaupapa, but all over, even on the outside. People sometimes think it is easier to let someone else do the job, maybe the dirty work, and then don't offer to pitch in, to say, "I know what you are doing, I support this, and we are behind you," even knowing that you have a solid base of confidence by vote, at Kalaupapa helps to keep me energized.

We are fighting for a principle, for our rights, for some basic human benefits. That's what the fight against the move from Hale Mohalu to Leahi is all about. No agency of Government has the right to fritter away our rights, our benefits, and our needs.

What made me take on the powerful State Government of Hawaii? Well, there have always been a lot of little local problems at Kalaupapa, with The Leprosy Program. I think some of those problems were told to you in four interviews at Kalaupapa. But I don't know if there was ever any straw that broke the camel's back, to set me off against the entire State of Hawaii administration. But all of a sudden I reached a point, due to the accumulation of injustices against us, I reached some point that set me off--as the elected representative of the patients. We can all go around nonchalantly not even realizing the things happening around you, then all of a sudden, bang, you realize there are a whole slew of things that have been committed against you. And all along, you have been a happy idiot! Just walking around, not knowing about these things.

I believe in the Constitution of the United States, and in the rights that each one of us has. When I see government agencies tell me and others that they are the government, they make decisions, and you as leprosy patients, because you are "wards" of the government, you must obey and you must be thankful. That . . . has always been contrary to my basic beliefs. The matter of obeying, following the dictates of the Hawaii State Health Department, and therefore you should be thankful for whatever we give you. Yes, I am thankful, but thankful that I have a Constitution with which to fight the injustices against us.

Over the years, the people of Kalaupapa, the leprosy patients in the State of Hawaii, have always had to fight injustices. Back in the middle 1860's, during Father Damien's time, in the 1900's, and today. Why is it that way? In 1978, someways, things are not too different from the 1940's or the late 1800's. Why it's like that is difficult to analyze. But it has gone full cycle, from the time when patients were torn away from their families and imprisoned at Kalawao peninsula. In those days, you obeyed! The concept of government was that, government knows what's best for you. And even today, that concept has not changed. Government's perception of leprosy patients, the perception of the Health Department especially, is that we are mindless. That we are zombies, incapable of thinking, of feeling. You know, this may be true not only in Hawaii, but maybe elsewhere. Government always seems to forget that they are the government of the people, for the people and by the people. Government is not some special thing, elevated to a high place. When government sees itself as being so high, they cease to function in our behalf.

I think leprosy patients are frightened to stand up and speak out, to fight for their rights. Many patients are frightened. It's not an easy thing. Because, when you have been dependent on the government, and when you have to challenge them on certain decisions, then the government starts to use pressures in many ways. And our people just crumble. In our case, the leprosy patients, intimidation goes back over one hundred years. We have been conditioned, we have been told, hey, do not do this, do not touch, do not breathe on other people. Do not associate. Visitors were advised to stay upwind of us in the old days. So that kind of conditioning makes our people shy. They avoid confronting the government. All their lives they have been dependent, and did what they were told to do. You can see why they are frightened to speak out. But me, I am not frightened. I think there is a definite tie-in with the Hale Mohalu issue and the future of Kalaupapa. If the Government can take Hale Mohalu away from us here at Pearl City, if they are successful, then they will be able to do practically the same thing at Kalaupapa. In spite of the fact that the legislature passed a bill, signed by the Governor, stating patients could live out the rest of their lives at Kalaupapa. Seeing the actions of the Hawaii State Government the last month, and the Governor's action, and the Health Department Director, they have all tried to undercut and discredit the Kalaupapa Advisory Council. Now, the Government advocates having a joint panel to determine what is best for the Kalaupapa community. People from the Land Department (Land and Natural Resources Department) Hawaiian Homes non-patient personnel, and some patients.

Another thing, it is amazing, though, we the Patients Council are elected by the Kalaupapa community—the Health Department says to the public at large, that we on the Kalaupapa patients council are not representative of the community of Kalaupapa on many issues. They make this statement public, and yet the Health Department has not done any survey to substantiate their claim. It's really amazing. (Re-elected 1-31-79)

Yes, people tell me I have come a long way. From being a patient inside Kalaupapa (I am still a patient there) to taking the leadership role for the patients, being more visible now in my role as spokesman for the patients. That is true. But I have one goal in mind. What I want to accomplish is simple. I want the State Government to realize something very basic about us as leprosy patients. They must realize we

110

have minds, we think, we love, we hate, we cry, you know . . . we rejoice. We have all the emotions and intellect of any person in society. And as such, to recognize that we are human. and thus extend to us the dignity that we are entitled to. It's not that we are granted dignity. Hey, this is something that everyone is born with. This is inherent in man's life, that he be accorded dignity. Not because he is some high official, a government figure who automatically acquires dignity, but because he is a person!

About unity among the Hawaiian people, at Kalaupapa, and within the State of Hawaii, sometimes you hear that the Hawaiians are not unified in this state. Well, that is true, and yet not true. I think there are certain groups now who share the same philosophy. Some Hawaiian groups in the Hawaii community can more easily rally around a goal. We see that with the Kahoolawe Ohana and other groups. But our community, at Kalaupapa, well, we have been isolated over the years, out of touch in many ways, and yet we are knowledgeable. Our people in the Kalaupapa community listen to the news, read newspapers, they know what is going on in the world. But I think the lack of interchange, lack of social intercourse, has not broadened our comprehension of events and how these events affect us. We have in our community, one of the most generous groups of people in the State of Hawaii. So many people marvel at the hospitality that is extended to them at Kalaupapa. But my one disappointment is that sometimes even in a family you have clashes of personality. Sometimes, with our people it is very difficult to put aside personal differences and rise above differences and fight for their own benefits. It seems like the only issue that would completely unite our people would be if there would be a threat of closing Kalaupapa. Many people say to me, "hey, we want you to represent us," yet some of these same people don't put in the time and effort to get involved, to help solve our problems. It is very difficult, for any in this position. Because I have been involved with the issues, and I have acquired some knowledge about the background on our issues, by that fact, I would hope our people would easily accept the knowledge and experience I have acquired. But it is very difficult to have this kind of acceptance, for a unified front.

The whole matter about the future of Kalaupapa has not been settled. There is much apprehension in Kalaupapa about our future. There are so many suggested uses for the community. Federal or National Park, State of Hawaii Park, County of Maui Park. Yet no decisions have been made. There are some good things about each potential use But I do know from my conversations with some Hawaii State legislators, that the State would not be in favor of having a National Park at Kalaupapa. One state legislator has said the State is not in the business of giving up land. They would not want to lose control of the land. I suppose that the State sees the potential for some resort development at Kalawao, down the road a piece. That's what I believe, because Governor Burns himself used to say it. He said, you would not believe the pressure that has been placed on us for resort development at Kalawao, to develop the area. And Governor Burns was truly a friend of ours. As long as he was in office, we were secure. I don't think this situation of forcing patients out of their Hale Mohalu Home would have developed if Governor Burns were still in office. We assumed that someone who shared the same administration would feel the same as our late governor, but I guess we were wrong.

Over the years, some of the main problems in the leprosy treatment program in Hawaii has been the matter of people's needs and wants versus physical structures. That is, land and buildings versus people's desires. The people at Kalaupapa, almost 90 percent want Hale Mohalu to remain as a treatment center in Honolulu, yet the State makes us move to another place we did not wish to go. The people wanted a new hospital for many years at Kalaupapa, yet they continued to keep an old fire trap as our hospital there. Only finally committed themselves to construction of a new hospital at Kalaupapa. Why is that? People's human wants and needs versus immaterial physical things. Physical things seem to be more important. People's needs and wants less important. Is that because of the stigma of leprosy or the nature of government? Government seeking profit above all, or is it a lack of sensitivity amongst leaders? I think it is a combination of all those things. Profit, or costs, seem to be the main criteria in the maintenance of the Hawaii leprosy program. At the University, I hear, anything they want, they can have. Also, the Governor has unlimited use of his

112

contingency funds and moves appropriations from A, to B, to C, and back to A again. In the end, I think the general public suffers.

You ask me, what I think the proper use of the Kalaupapa peninsula would be, because we have a declining population at Kalaupapa. I'm inclined to think that we should consider a gradual relaxation of people permitted into the settlement. Make it easier to get in, not the general public, but easier for the families of leprosy patients to get in. Maybe you could start with these family members, to allow them to reside with their leprosy family within Kalaupapa. That would be an ideal situation. For instance, as long as I remain at Kalaupapa, maybe my mother could come and live with me, but at no expense to the State, should she become a widow. At least that way families could have some kind of relationship with each other. Again, not at the expense of the state. I'm not saying that everyone would want this. This kind of thinking might seem too radical from the kind of thinking we have been accustomed to, the isolation and all we have experienced over the years. But I would rather see our family members brought into the community, rather than have the community geared exclusively as a tourist mecca. There is no doubt that because of the historical significance of Father Damien's place of work and death, his church, people come from all over the world because of the heroics of this man. They come there to see the land, the Aina, where he had given of his life. That seems to be inevitable, but I think there should be some control, there should be no carte blanche invasion of tourists into Kalaupapa.

Some people have mentioned the possibility of Kalaupapa becoming an international research and treatment center for leprosy work, in keeping with the heroic deeds of Damien and the people he served, the courageous people who lived and died there since the 1860's, but also to take into account the pride and dignity of the ancient Hawaiian culture which existed in Kalawao before Kalaupapa was established for leprosy patients. Some international authorities in leprosy treatment have expressed an interest in this kind of idea, the research community at Kalaupapa. But I am not sure that would work. An international research station, with

113

our patients and maybe other patients from the Pacific and Southeast Asia, would be a hard thing to put together. You know, the main trend today is to have patients live in the outside community. To 'mainstream' them. The other thing is that the land game is important. This is very important land, and the state wants it. The land game is always in the forefront. But the idea of confining people for research purposes has become foreign to modern medical thinking. And I favor that, because I know what it was like to be confined. To be imprisoned. That is exactly what happened, what it was. I was forbidden to even touch my mother, my brother, my sister, my family. When they used to come visit me at Kalihi Hospital, they were only a few feet away from me, but it might have been a thousand miles. Because we couldn't touch. I can remember my brother and sister running through the gate of the hospital, and being yelled at by the matron who was in charge of the hospital, I still can remember vividly what it was like. It hurts sometimes.

Maybe I have traveled a long road from that time of confinement to my leadership role today. But, you know, it is not something I have sought, this leadership. I can be a very good follower. But, sometimes I feel like saying, let someone else come in and take this role. Let somebody else try out their abilities. But, sometimes you get frustrated, because some of our people don't want to participate in decisions that affect their lives, to take leadership and fight for their rights. But maybe that is what keeps me going. I still don't like people making decisions for me. I have never been the kind who says, "Yes, thank you boss." "Thank you Mr. Superintendent, thank you Mr. Doctor." I used to get punished at Kalaupapa when I was a young kid, because I spoke up. So, bang, sometimes I couldn't go to the movies as my punishment. And the movies were everything to me. There was nothing else to do. Or get punished for having dirty fingernails. When you had dirty fingernails, you got it on your butt.

There is a contradiction among us, that maybe you know about. We get 1.4 million dollars a year for the leprosy treatment program in Hawaii. Most of our people express satisfaction with the medical treatment they get inside

114

Kalaupapa. Although they are not for the forced eviction of us from Hale Mohalu to Leahi, they do express satisfaction with their medical treatment. Yet, some doctors, leprologists, in the mainland, say we do not get good treatment for the money the state receives. International leprologists have criticized Hawaii's treatment program. Why do our patients express satisfaction, yet some outside specialists express criticism of our program? It's because of how our people are, like I said before. We go back to the very beginning when Kalaupapa was born. The birth of Kalaupapa. From that moment, until even today, our patients accept. You know what it is? It is that respect for authority. Just recently a gentleman told me that. He is in his eighties. This is ingrained in us. There is humility and respect among our people, so sometimes they do not say what they really have on their minds. And they don't realize the quality of care available elsewhere, like Carville.

Myself, I am not awed by authority. If a person respects me, I respect them. Whether they hold the position of Senator, Representative, janitor, it don't matter. I'm not awed by any position. My friendship does not lie in the kind of position a person holds. I take each individual on their character. If we hit it off, great. It can be the guy digging the ditch. I used to dig ditch, myself. But I think our people are very polite. They do not want to offend the doctor, or the bureaucrat, the administrator, even if we are getting short-changed. For years, the officials have told us, let's not rock the boat, let's not ask for too much from the Federal Government from the Health Education and Welfare. Maybe if we do ask for more, they will give us less. Let's not ask for too much from the Legislature either. Don't complain too much. If you do, they may come in and do things we are going to be sorry for. We may have it worse, not better. And I have heard our people say this. "Don't, Don't," they say. "Don't ask for that." "Keep it quiet." "Be careful!" I can remember one lady said, "No ask for too much thing," she told me. I said, "Hey, if you need it, we ask for it."

If I were in charge of the leprosy program in Hawaii, at Kalaupapa and in the state, what ten improvements would I make? Well, there are many. First of all, I would get rid of the career bureaucrats. Those who have made a living off our ailment. These same people, even after twenty or thirty years, have never developed any sensitivity to our needs and feelings. No sensitivity to the people they are supposed to care for. I would get rid of the Department Heads who have been dealing with us, starting with the Director of Health, who have no background in Public Health or Medicine. I would see that whoever sits in the position has some background in medicine or at least in Public Health. Certainly not a Civil Engineer. And I would appoint administrators who would allow patients to participate in real decision making, participate in decisions that affect their lives. Real decisions. Real opportunity to participate in policy and administrative decisions.

There are many things we need in the community. For many years, we have needed a fire truck. We have had no fire protection for years. Not only this, this old fire truck we have doesn't run, it runs, but it must be pushed to start, and the water pump does not work. So it is useless. And our buildings are old, old, and made of wood. For years we have asked for a fire truck that works. But the Dept. of Health's main approach has been to try and cut off what they can from the community; to save money. Always they see what they can cut back, even our fire protection. We need a new water tank due to the constant breakage in our waterline, five or six times a year, along the coastline, which requires rationing of water. Another example. Our chlorinator is an old one. Our water gets contaminated with too much bacteria. It must be boiled to make it safe for drinking. Now this is hard for the old people, especially those with twisted hands and no feelings in their fingers. But quite often they must boil all of their water, because the old chlorinator keeps breaking down. Finally, after many years, the Dept. of Health purchased a new chlorinator. But then, someone fixed the old one. So, the new chlorinator was not used, or maybe returned. Instead they used the money for something else. Then, wouldn't you know it, the old chlorinator broke again. So again, this summer in 1978, the old folks have had to boil their water. Things have gone on like that for years. The damn old chlorinator. Those are the kind of decisions that we always suffer from.

Also, we need a dialysis unit at Kalaupapa. Many of our people have kidney problems, but there is no trained specialist with a dialysis unit within our community to help our people. Our people must go to Honolulu to get their treatment. Finally, after years and years, they tell us we will finally get our kidney unit at Kalaupapa. It will be in the new clinic they are building. But of course, we have also needed a new clinic for many years. I think they just try to hold back monies, funds, from us. It's kind of a race between us, aging patients, and time, and the old buildings. Who will give out, what will give out first? All the while, they save their money--money that was appropriated from the HEW to help us leprosy patients.

There are so many things which must be done. So many. Again, repair the existing old buildings. Roofs leak. Buildings need painting, both in the individual patients' quarters and in McVeigh Hall. The Hall is important because it is used for patient meetings and luaus. The hole in the roof is so large, you can see the stars through it at night. Of course, it leaks very bad when it rains.

Of paramount importance is a resident physician. We have not had a full-time doctor at Kalaupapa for about three years. We have had a doctor serving about 130 patients about fourteen hours a week. Two days a week, about seven hours per day. We have had two or three deaths within Kalaupapa, within the last two years, without a physician in attendance Again, maybe we don't have a doctor because they want to save money. The Director says "we're looking for a Doctor." But he knows damn well, they cut off the position from Kalaupapa. Why do they have to lie to us?

Overall, what we need most, are administrators who care for us. Administrators who care for us as human beings. The ones now, they seem more interested in collecting their paychecks. We need professionals managing our programs, not political appointees. We need doctors, public health specialists, managing our program, not political people. There is so much we need. So much to be done.

There are a few things that I'd like to do for myself, like attending the University of Hawaii, and also, try to get my song compositions recorded and published. And perhaps to give politics a try. But, at this point in time, Patients Rights has a higher priority, and those things will keep for a while on the back burner. Some, who know my medical problems have suggested that I go to Carville (the U.S. Public Health Leprosarium in Louisiana) to care for them. But, while the idea is intriguing, I am afraid to leave. If I don't speak out for my people, who will? I cannot afford the luxury of a respite from this mission. I have pledged total commitment to the struggle of Hale Mohalu and Kalaupapa, in attaining human rights and dignity for all of us.

AFTERWORD—FATHER DAMIEN'S LEGACY

Father Damien, Joseph De Veuster, was a healthy and robust Belgian missionary priest of the Sacred Hearts Fathers. He volunteered for service in Hawaii and, after arriving, asked to serve as the Catholic missionary at Kalaupapa. Father Damien died at Kalaupapa on April 15, 1889, after contracting leprosy in the course of his sixteen years among the patients there. His service stands as an example of one man's acute awareness, sensitivity, and dedication to the needs of leprosy patients.

Although Father Damien's life and death brought him worldwide attention and acclaim, this fame was often an embarrassment and source of consternation to his clerical superiors and to the Board of Health administrators in Honolulu.

Gavin Daws, author of Holy Man, explains the reason for this discomfiture among his superiors. Father Damien was an unorthodox priest, a man of unrestrained dedication, with an exuberance for his patients and his work among them. He was charismatic, individualistic, and impatient with authority; surrounded by his own "personal turbulence of holiness." Though Father Damien gave his life to assist the helpless, close to home officials thought him a troublemaker.

This discrepancy between the laudatory world view of the man and the more narrow local political-official damnation of him may be his legacy. Further this discrepancy may have been carried over to this day to be borne by others like him, the contemporary leprosy patients active as social activists on behalf of patients' rights. Then as now, the vested interest politics of the state government and the Health Department have not been especially sympathetic to the needs of leprosy patients.

The distance of time provides a better view of martyrs, and today Father Damien's record of martyrdom, sacrifice, and personal mortification has resulted in his candidacy for sainthood. In Hawaii, Damien's date of death is an official day of rememberance. A powerful rendering of the man (a statue by Marisol Escobar) stands before the Hawaii State Capitol building in Honolulu; a duplicate is enshrined in Washington, D.C. In Hawaii, on Father Damien's Day children decorate his statue with flower leis and high school bands (there is one school bearing his name) march by in parade, trumpeting in pride. But Damien's legacy is not measured in statues and school holidays. He represents much more than the accolades in speeches by state officials on congratulatory days of latent good intentions, the celebration of goodness after the fact.

Leprosy patients will be embarrassed by our saying so, but today there are individuals doing Father Damien-like work. They are the leprosy patients themselves, struggling with illness, and for the dignity of their civil rights. This struggle is expressed in the preceding interview titled "The Time Capsule," in which the patient suggests that nothing has changed since Father Damien's time. Just as Damien fought against the obstacles of his own illness and the administrative indifference shown him and his fellow patients, so, too, modern leprosy patient leaders struggle. And like Father Damien, they also have received worldwide acclaim, attention and support from the media and international church groups. Locally, they continue to be the recipients of government indifference, neglect, and the butt of official power used against them.

The forcible eviction of the leprosy patients from their old home, Hale Mohalu, prompted the United States Federal Judge Shirley Hufsteadler to comment that Hawaii's leprosy patients have suffered "the reprehensible and unconscionable actions of the State of Hawaii." The State evicted the patients from their Pearl City "half-way house"—although they were long-time residents of the place—and charged the elderly and disabled with trespass. The State then went on to shut off the water, cut the electric wires supplying current to the facility, halt food, medical, nursing and other life support services to these dependent people, who, for the first time in their lives, were attempting to take a public stand on their own behalf. All these actions were taken while the patients' attorneys were legally contesting the eviction with the state and federal court systems. Reprehensible and unconscionable indeed!

On the day of eviction, police helicopters circled overhead; State police with high powered sidearms entered the old hospital to remove and arrest patients and their supporters. Outside, bulldozers stood ready to demolish the building moments after the patients were forcibly removed. Those who did not have time to rescue their belongings, watched them being crushed by the machines. Even Father Damien did not have to endure a "military" action.

In an Orwellian twist, the large hospital ward to which the patients were removed had been renamed earlier the "Hale Mohalu at Leahi Hospital." Let this story be told by the politicians on Father Damien's Day!

Finally, a word about the future of the people of Kalaupapa. They are safe. A congressional law was passed in 1980 to establish the Kalaupapa National Historical Park; under federal protection, the Kalaupapa residents are guaranteed the right to remain in residence at their community for as long as they wish. There will be no evictions, no construction of hotels, golf courses or other development inconsistent with the history of the place. The National Park Service has promised to preserve and interpret Kalaupapa for present and future generations.

Ted Gugelyk

EPILOGUE

Kalaupapa is no longer a place of forced incarceration. A new chapter of its history has begun. But its past still haunts us. Memories of Kalaupapa as a place of imprisonment (forced domicile, if you prefer) for thousands of people sick with leprosy will always remain. After all, men, women, and children were hunted down; bounties were placed on their heads as if they were criminals; and they were left to die there—for the greater good of society. Those few who remain (approximately sixty eight in 1996) are remnants of that tragic time. They are the survivors of those whose lives were sacrificed for societies well-being. Quarantine was the method used world wide in dealing with the disease. The sacrifices the leprosy patients were forced to make are both heroic and tragic. No memorial, testimonial, or official proclamation of gratitude can lessen the personal pain of these survivors. Their memories are seared by their past. Yet ironically, what was once their prison is now their cherished home. They wish to remain at Kalaupapa until they die. And why not? It is a beautiful, peaceful place, a place of refuge from the increasingly urbanized life of contemporary Hawaii.

Kalaupapa is now a National Park, a protected place. Thousands of tourists visit each year, and many more will come in the future—especially now that Father Damien has been canonized by the Catholic Church. Part of Father Damien's has been returned from Belgium to Kalaupapa, to repose among the people he loved and served. His place of burial will become a kind of shrine and memorial to his good works. And fittingly so.

Unfortunately, in this life there are other Kalaupapas, other places where innocents are incarcerated, persecuted, tortured and killed—sometimes because of another kind of sickness, a sickness in man's soul. I am thinking, of course, of the holocausts, the concentration and extermination camps of World War II, and the camps in Bosnia and Herzegovina, Cambodia, Vietnam, and Africa—places unrelated geographically but the closest of kin in brutal cruelty and injustice. There is a common denominator here. It is a lack of compassion. The most powerless, the most vulnerable, are the first to be incarcerated, the first to die. That was Father Damien's concern. That is why Kalaupapa is so important in Hawaii's history. It was a place where both cruelty and compassion existed, side by side.

The authors of this book formed a small foundation to publish their work. They wanted to preserve some of the patients' stories about their lives at Kalaupapa. Most of the patients whose lives are recounted here have since died. But their personal experiences remain powerful and compelling reading. We hope that this small book will continue to be read by people interested in Kalaupapa's history. This is now the third edition of the The Separating Sickness. Interest in Kalaupapa's history and future still continues.

We have never realized a profit from this work; all monies gained have been used to publish updated editions of the book. If we ever do realize a profit, part of that profit will be used for acts of benevolence. Leprosy is still a problem world wide. Although modern medication seems to have it under control, it still afflicts many millions of people. And, although mandatory confinement of newly diagnosed leprosy suffers is no longer an accepted social policy anywhere, leprosy patients still suffer from a powerful stigma, even in developed nations. In Japan, in 1996, the nation maintains fifteen leprosariums that house approximately five thousand patients. Although these patients venture out into society, they do so at their own risk. Prejudice and hostility against them is still strong in Japan—and, indeed, in most of Asia. In fact there is still an archaic Japanese law that forbids patients to leave their isolated leprosarium grounds. According to a recent Associated Press story, a bill that would officially allow Japanese patients to return to society was introduced in the Japanese parliament in February 1996. It was expected to pass and thus to end—at last— a system under which more than thirty thousand people were condemned to isolation.

I am especially interested in the children of leprosy patients living in the less developed nations of the world. Leprosy is a disease that afflicts the poor and those living in unhygienic conditions, and there are many millions of them. Children of the poor are always the most vulnerable. I have seen such children in Cambodia and Vietnam. Their situation is desperate. Their nations are among the poorest in the world, although, with international assistance, they are trying hard to improve conditions as they recover from generations of devastating warfare. Gifts of simple things such as clothes, books, and pencils would mean a lot. If this book should generate a profit, we shall use part of it to help the children of leprosy patients.

Ted Gugelyk